In Search of Dignity

In Search of Dignity

A Lifetime of Reflections

HARVEY MAX CHOCHINOV

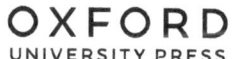

OXFORD
UNIVERSITY PRESS

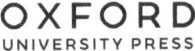

Oxford University Press is a department of the University of Oxford.
It furthers the University's objective of excellence in research, scholarship,
and education by publishing worldwide. Oxford is a registered trade mark of
Oxford University Press in the UK and in certain other countries.

Published in the United States of America by Oxford University Press
198 Madison Avenue, New York, NY 10016, United States of America.

CIP data is on file at the Library of Congress

ISBN 9780197805114

DOI: 10.1093/9780197805145.001.0001

Printed by Integrated Books International, United States of America

The manufacturer's authorized representative in the EU for product safety is
Oxford University Press España S.A. of Parque Empresarial San Fernando de Henares,
Avenida de Castilla, 2 – 28830 Madrid (www.oup.es/en or product.safety@oup.com).
OUP España S.A. also acts as importer into Spain of products made by the manufacturer.

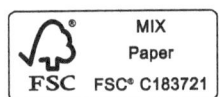

The manufacturer's authorised representative in the EU for product safety is Oxford University Press España S.A. of El Parque Empresarial
San Fernando de Henares, Avenida de Castilla, 2 – 28830 Madrid (www.oup.es/en or product.safety@oup.com). OUP España S.A. also acts as
importer into Spain of products made by the manufacturer.

In memory of my mother, Shirley Chochinov, and my sister, Ellen Chochinov
For Michelle, Lauren, Rachel, and Cam
And my grandson, Riley Maddox Marr

Contents

SECTION 4. REFLECTIONS ON HASTENING DEATH

SECTION 5. PERSONAL REFLECTIONS

Introduction

The thought of writing a conventional biography doesn't entice me. It's not only that I suspect few people would find it of interest, but rather, it just doesn't spark my creative imagination. On the other hand, writing a *vocational biography*—that is, a candid and nostalgic reflection on various facets of my medical career—now that feels intriguing. And why is that the case and why might anyone care?

To be frank, these past four decades have taken me on a professional journey beyond anything I could ever have imagined. This quest—and I call it that, realizing in hindsight I was looking for something—began in Winnipeg, Canada, at the University of Manitoba, where I completed my core training in medicine and psychiatry. This led to the hallowed halls of Cornell Medical College and Memorial Sloan Kettering Cancer Center in New York City. With Winnipeg as my home base, I forged research collaborations with colleagues worldwide, including medical luminaries on several continents. Each study, each paper, each book, each student, and each lecture in academic institutions around the globe have helped me shape areas of medicine most dear to my heart—palliative care and person-centered care.

In Search of Dignity: A Lifetime of Reflections is a collection of publications and speeches I've penned over the years. Each one is accompanied by contemporary musings, telling the story behind the story and what motivated me to write that piece, or how my words currently resonate, considering shifting social policies and medical practices over time. The book is divided into five sections: *Early Beginnings, Dignity . . . and More Dignity, Personhood and Attending to Suffering, Reflections on Hastening Death*, and *Personal Reflections*. With hundreds to choose from, I decided not to include papers that were data driven; those tend to be more technical in nature and can be found in peer-reviewed journals. On the other hand, I selected "think pieces"; essays, newspaper articles, and speeches reflecting my thoughts on topics that felt relevant at the time.

In Search of Dignity: A Lifetime of Reflections explores issues I've grappled with my entire career, issues that strike at the heart of what it means to be human, to be vulnerable, and to be mortal. Although my clinical and

In Search of Dignity. Harvey Max Chochinov, Oxford University Press. © Oxford University Press 2025.
DOI: 10.1093/9780197805145.001.0001

academic work has focused on palliative care, the insights I've acquired these past four decades resonate across the entirety of life. In a career that has fostered humility and enlightenment, patients have revealed the kind of wisdom that becomes most transparent in proximity to death. In hindsight, I think they gave me exactly what I was looking for. This book is my opportunity to share that with you.

SECTION 1
EARLY BEGINNINGS

1

The Culture of Research in Palliative Care

You Probably Think This Song Is About You

Throughout my career, Dr. Eduardo Bruera has been an inspiration and role model. His contributions to the field of palliative care are prolific. Besides his legendary prowess as a scholar and clinician–scientist, he is a polyglot and avid runner. Here is the speech I gave in 2015 upon receiving an award named in his honor.

* * * * *

As one of the few psychiatrists in the crowd, I thought I would provide some deep psychological reflections on what this award means to me, and what issues it has stirred up. Since winning the Eduardo Bruera Award in Palliative Medicine, I have had the irresistible urge to learn French, Spanish, Portuguese, German, and Italian. Considering his athletic prowess, I also find myself looking in the mirror occasionally with disdain, thinking that perhaps I should work out more, loose a few pounds, kick my pathetic exercise routine up a notch or two. I admit, I have looked at Scopus and discovered that my number of indexed articles, about 140 not counting books and chapters (which bring it to about 200)—and total citations—about 5,500, seem a mere pittance to Eduardo's astronomical 800 articles and just over 22,000 career citations![a]When he was in Edmonton at the start of my career, I loved reminding myself, by way of his example, that people make a place great and not the other way around. I've always admired him; but he has set the bar so high that looking up to him these last 25 years or so has started to strain my neck. I remember once presenting at a meeting with Eduardo, and our host went around the conference room table, introducing each of us in turn. When he got to Eduardo he said, "and this is Dr. Bruera—he is the king." So, perhaps winning this award makes me the Little Prince.

My favorite quote from The Little Prince *by Antoine de Saint-Exupery reads, "A rock pile ceases to be a rock pile the moment a single man*

---

[a] In 2025, I have 355 articles with 28,000 citations; Eduardo has over 1,800 articles with a stunning 87,000 citation!

In Search of Dignity. Harvey Max Chochinov, Oxford University Press. © Oxford University Press 2025. DOI: 10.1093/9780197805145.003.0001

contemplates it, bearing within him the image of a cathedral." That is the kind of thinking Eduardo Bruera has encouraged in our field; seeing what is and using research as a bridge towards creating something better. As you may recall, the Little Prince spoke in parables and poetry and so shall I.

And the Little Prince asked: "Your Majesty, what is the secret of your success?"

And the King responded, "Hypodermoclysis."[b]

The Little Prince was puzzled, uncertain of the wisdom hidden therein.

And the King explained, "Research is a long and difficult journey; you need to be focused, you need to be persistent, and you need to keep well hydrated."

"And, Your Majesty, how will I know if I am on the right path?"

To which the King responded, "Opioid rotation."[c] And again, the Little Prince was confused. The King explained, "If, after a while, studying the same thing is making you feel crazy, don't be afraid to switch things around."

And finally, the Little Prince asked the most difficult question of all: "Your Majesty, in this Eduardian kingdom, you have cast a long shadow. How will I know when I have done enough? How will I know when I am worthy of stepping beyond your shadow and into the sunlight?"

To which the King responded, "Euthanasia."

The Little Prince was befuddled.

The King explained, "Your insecurity and tiresome questions are boring me to death. Just accept the damn award; people are hungry and want to get on with dinner."

To which the Little Prince, turning to the audience, said, "Thank you, merci, gracias, obrigato, danke, grazie."

* * * * *

When I first launched my program of palliative care research in 1990, I invited Dr. Bruera to Winnipeg to speak with our staff and get them excited about studies involving patients nearing end of life. This article describes a very specific encounter that took place during his visit, which has stayed with me ever since.

---

[b] A method of administering fluids or medication under the skin.

[c] A switch from one opioid to another to improve the response to analgesic therapy or reduce adverse effects.

The Culture of Research in Palliative Care: You Probably Think This Song Is About You. Harvey Max Chochinov. *Journal of Palliative Medicine,* 2009;12(3):215–217. Reprinted with permission from Mary Ann Liebert, Inc. publishers.

"But is it right?"

If my memory can be trusted, the question came after a presentation by *the* Eduardo Bruera on the importance of research in palliative care. I believe it was the fall of 1990 and Dr. Bruera was in Winnipeg to help launch my first study. The nurse asking this question—and no, I do not remember who it was—did so, not in a way that felt dismissive or punitive, but rather, with a sense of genuine caring and concern. After all, people approaching death have limited time and energy. Did we really want to be asking them, indeed, was it right to be asking them to expend effort in answering our research questions?[1] Many have argued that the terminally ill are vulnerable and ought to be protected from enrollment in research studies,[2,3] given they are unlikely to realize any advantage in return for their loss of time and energy.[4] I clearly remember Dr. Bruera's response—one that rings as true today as it did so many years ago. In essence, he asked if the status quo was worth defending. In other words, were we convinced that the quality of care, the efficacy of treatment and the completeness of knowledge underpinning palliative care were beyond reproach or the possibility of improvement? If so, there was neither justification nor cause to proceed. On the other hand, if care for the dying is less than optimal—whether in reference to the physical, psychological, psychosocial, spiritual, or existential challenges facing patients and families confronting life-threatening or life-limiting conditions—how can we morally justify not doing palliative care research?

For years I have thought about that question and Dr. Bruera's response (perhaps it was a physician, a social worker, or maybe a spiritual care provider who asked the question; it's hard to recall). Ever since then, I think about the status quo in terms of how things are today, and research in terms of the promise for tomorrow. It is an inspiring credo and, for me, one that has made palliative care research ethically comfortable. Appropriately, the literature has stressed how this comfort must be achieved within an ethical framework that balances the demands of research with acceptable protocol burden and risk.[1] Patient vulnerability can also be heightened by minority status, poverty, lack of health insurance, diminished capacity, or other causes of lacking a voice. For these reasons, protectionism has defined the culture of institutional ethics boards and to varying degrees, the attitudes of palliative care clinicians. While research is important, the individual needs of patients and families must always take precedence, and participants carefully selected and respectfully shielded.

But long since that inimitable *Eduardian* response, experience in palliative care research has revealed another important truth. While we have worried about protocol burden—researchers, ethics review boards and clinicians alike—participants facing life-limiting circumstances have willingly and often enthusiastically enrolled in our studies. Those not too sick (the major reason for non-participation) and able to squeeze past the "gatekeepers"[5,6]— well-intentioned individuals wanting to shield patients from harm—have answered questions and provided insights into the broadest range of issues imaginable: what is it like to feel vulnerable?[7]; what defines your sense of dignity?[8-10]; are you depressed?[11,12]; tell me about your distress?[13]; do you ever find yourself wishing life was over?[14,15]; tell me about what suffering means to you?[16,17] These are not easy questions. Yet, after nearly 20 years of asking patients and families about the intimate details of confronting death, the legions of damaged, distressed or disgruntled participants have not materialized. Oh, perhaps a handful (no more) have indicated some minor distress or irritation, but nothing that has required anything beyond basic clarification or simple reassurance.

However, an even more profound insight has begun to dawn since Eduardo spoke so eloquently that day in Winnipeg about moral justice and palliative care research (perhaps it wasn't Winnipeg? . . . could it have been London, Paris, Tokyo or Barcelona?—my, how memory fades). That is, not only don't participants feel distressed, they seem to like and benefit from taking part in research. My first inkling of this began years ago, when we started asking patients about their desire for early death.[14,15] Rather than being spurned or rebuffed, patients often thanked us for broaching "the unspeakable," for providing an opportunity to talk about feelings that others did not want to address or were unable to hear. During a recent randomized control trial, even patients and families assigned to the non-intervention arm would often express appreciation for being able to answer baseline questions about their distress and coping. (Given this was an RCT, you can imagine how much good this did my heart!)

Others have begun to examine the flipside of "research as burden." Among a cohort of 68 patients with end-stage cancer, the vast majority reported no burden partaking in psychosocial research; most found the experience moderately to highly beneficial.[18] Factors associated with burden included the length of the interview (21%), structure of the questionnaires (18%), and discussing end-of-life issues (12%); only 4 patients (6%) felt the research was significantly burdensome, although none dropped out of the study. The most common reported benefits included enjoying the social interaction (75%), feeling a sense of contribution to society (57%), helping to keep them busy (47%), and the therapeutic gain of being able to discuss their illness at length (43%). The overwhelming majority (77%) stated that they would agree to participate again if given the opportunity. It has also been reported that research is well accepted by participants in specialist palliative care units. Of 40 patients with advanced stages of illness, two thirds were quite happy or very happy to be involved in research trials, although studies that were more physically invasive were perceived to be more burdensome.[19] In a study of nearly 1000 patients taking part in end-of-life discussions, fewer than 2% experienced a great deal of stress, 7.1% some stress, and 88.7% little or no stress.[20] Nearly half (46.5%) the patients and slightly more caregivers (53.4%) felt their participation had been somewhat or very helpful. Notably, 61% of patients who reported fear, anxiety, or difficulty with issues of closure found the interview especially helpful. Seamark[21] conducted post-death interviews with 79 family members, 2 months after the death of their loved one. Eighty-three percent of participants reported no to mild distress and three quarters rated the interview as helpful to very helpful.

To be clear, the culture of palliative care research has evolved. While these studies were once considered dubious and even morally suspect, those times appear to be behind us. Perhaps the notion of palliative care research as a "burdensome necessity" will segue to an appreciation of its potential as a therapeutic opportunity. As a wise research colleague recently pointed out, "Some patients even appreciate being given the chance to turn down a research study" (K. Cullihall, personal communication, September 2008). This does not mean that protective gates for vulnerable populations are not necessary, to a degree, but the danger of building those gates too high denies patients and families the opportunity to make autonomous, self-determined choices about participating in research.[5,6] Patients who sense they have limited time often find solace in knowing their contribution will promote the advancement of science.[23] Little wonder that the vast majority of seriously ill patients rank being able to help others as one of five top items they valued at the end of life.[24] The salutary effects of taking part in research may very well be the enhanced sense of meaning and purpose that provides the foundation of dignity-conserving care.[25]

Eduardo: Harvey, to be honest, I don't remember anything about making those particular comments.

Harvey: Come on, you've got to be kidding me!

Eduardo: Nope, I'm afraid not. I entirely agree with those statements, I'm just saying I don't remember making them. By the way, I like the way you make me sound really smart.

Harvey: Eduardo, you *are* really smart. I suppose this means you have no idea who asked that question about the moral justification of palliative care research?

Eduardo: No. But you and I both know, pretty much anyone, anywhere might have sung that particular tune.

For those of you with "one eye in the mirror," I can only say that Eduardo still has a way of pushing aside those "clouds in his coffee," placing his finger squarely on the truth.

References

1. Field MJ, Cassel CK. *Approaching Death: Improving Care at the End of Life.* National Academy Press; 1997.
2. Annas GJ. The changing landscape of human experimentation: Nuremberg, Helsinki, and beyond. *Health Matrix.* 1992;2:119–139.
3. Cassel C. Ethical issues in the conduct of research in long term care. *Gerontologist.* 1998;28(suppl):S90–S96.
4. Wilkie P. Ethical issues in qualitative research in palliative care. In: Field D, Clark D, Corner J, David C, eds. *Researching Palliative Care.* Open University Press; 2001:67–74.
5. Addington-Hall J. Research sensitivities to palliative care patients. *Eur J Cancer Care.* 2002;11;220–224.
6. Janssens R, Gordijn B. Clinical trial in palliative care: an ethical evaluation. *Patient Educ Couns.* 2000;41:55–62.
7. Stienstra D, Chochinov HM. Vulnerability, disability and palliative end-of-life care. *J Palliat Care.* 2006;22:166–174.
8. Chochinov HM. Dignity-conserving care: a new model for palliative care. *JAMA.* 2002;287:2253–2260.
9. Chochinov HM, Hack T, McClement S, et al. Dignity in the terminally ill: a developing empirical model. *Soc Sci Med.* 2002;54:433–443.
10. Chochinov HM, Hack T, Hassard T, et al. Dignity in the terminally ill: a cross-sectional, cohort study. *Lancet.* 2002;360:2026–2030.

11. Chochinov HM, Wilson K, Enns M, Lander S. Are you depressed? Screening for depression in the terminally ill. *Am J Psychiatry.* 1997;154:674–676.

12. Chochinov HM, Wilson KG, Enns M, Lander S. The prevalence of depression in the terminally ill: effects of diagnostic criteria and symptom threshold judgments. *Am J Psychiatry.* 1994;151:4.

13. Chochinov HM, Hassard T, McClement S, et al. The patient dignity inventory: a novel way of measuring dignity-related distress in palliative care. *J Pain Symptom Manage.* 2008;36:559–571.

14. Chochinov HM, Wilson KG, Enns M, et al. Desire for death in the terminally ill. *Am J Psychiatry.* 1995;152:1185–1191.

15. Chochinov HM, Tataryn D, Dudgeon D, Clinch J. Will to live in the terminally ill. *Lancet.* 1999;354:816–819.

16. Wilson K, Chochinov HM, McPherson C, et al. Suffering with advanced cancer. *J Clin Oncol.* 2007;25:1691–1697.

17. Chochinov HM, Kristjanson L, Hack T, et al. Burden to others and the terminally ill. *J Pain Symptom Manage.* 2007;34:463–471.

18. Pessin H, Galietta M, Nelson CJ, et al. Burden and benefit of psychosocial research at the end of life. *J Palliat Med.* 2008;11:627–632.

19. Ross C, Cornbleet M. Attitudes of patients and staff to research in a specialist palliative care unit. *Palliat Med.* 2003;17:491–497.

20. Emanuel EJ, Fairclough DL, Wolfe P, Emanuel LL. Talking with terminally ill patients and their caregivers about death, dying, and bereavement: Is it stressful? Is it helpful? *Arch Intern Med.* 2004;164:1999–2004.

21. Seamark DA. Are post-bereavement research interviews distressing to carers? Lessons learned from palliative care research. *Palliat Med.* 2000;14:55–56.

22. Ling J, Rees E, Harding J. What influences participation in clinical trials in palliative care in a cancer center? *Eur J Cancer.* 2000;36:621–626.

23. Steinhauser KE, Christakis NA, Clipp EC, et al. Factors considered important at the end of life by patients, family, physicians, and other care providers. *JAMA.* 2000;284:2476–2482.

24. Chochinov HM. Dignity and the essence of medicine: the A, B, C and D of dignity-conserving care. *BMJ.* 2007;335:184–187.

2

The Five Research C's

It was never my intent to become a researcher. My fellowship at Memorial Sloan Kettering left me utterly disinclined to do so. My mentors there were incredible, each leaders in their field. But they seemed to be driven, trying to abide by too many taskmasters, one telling them to be consummate clinicians, another reminding them they were first and foremost teachers, and one goading them to do cutting-edge research. No matter how they spent their days—seeing patients on the wards, mentoring trainees, or putting the final touches on their grants or papers—I always got the impression they saw themselves failing to fulfill their various sacred obligations. Which is why, upon returning to Winnipeg, Canada, in 1987, I was perfectly content to immerse myself in clinical work. I helped establish a Department of Psychosocial Oncology at the Manitoba Cancer Treatment and Research Foundation and spent most of my time seeing patients.

One fateful day, circa 1990, our clinical team reviewed an article by Dr. James Brown et al. entitled "Is It Normal for Terminally Ill Patients to Desire Early Death?" (Am J Psychiatry. 1986;143:208–211). There were many things about the article that made me curious and led me to ponder various questions needing answers. I immediately made my way to the office of Dr. Keith Wilson, a psychologist who'd been hired by the Department of Psychiatry to encourage staff to consider doing clinical research. With Keith as my gifted mentor, we assembled a research application that within 2 months was funded. That was about 35 years ago. Since then, no two workdays have felt alike. Conducting research has been and remains intellectually invigorating, personally fulfilling, and deeply meaningful. And the cyclical nature of research—questions leading to answers, leading to more questions—led me to write about the "Five Research C's."

In Search of Dignity. Harvey Max Chochinov, Oxford University Press. © Oxford University Press 2025.
DOI: 10.1093/9780197805145.003.0002

The Five Research C's. Harvey Max Chochinov. *Palliative & Supportive Care,* 2007;5(3):203–205. Reproduced with permission from Cambridge University Press.

It is naïve to think that successful research, like any lifelong academic pursuit, can be reduced to a pithy, simplistic formula. Yet, after years of attempting to get it right and with still much to learn, it strikes me that successful research is comprised of certain indispensable elements. Based on considerable personal experience and reflection, I humbly offer the "Five Research C's"; their intent is to provide a framework for novice and expert investigators alike, to contemplate some of the basic elements of empirical research.

Curiosity: Without curiosity, there is no research; it's as simple as that. Questions are the essence of research, and it takes curiosity to generate those all-important questions. There is nothing more coveted by researchers than questions that intrigue, questions that generate intellectual excitement, questions that grab hold and simply will not let go. Questions such as these make looking for answers worthy of immense effort. The person whose curiosity elicits questions of this caliber brings the most precious of commodities to the research endeavor. The questions and methods used to answer them need not be elaborate. But questions, even straightforward, seemingly simple questions, can make for very fine research.

As a rather wonderful case in point, sometime in the early 1880s, one of the early "microbe hunters," Robert Koch, noticed several different colored droplets scattered on the surface of a half, boiled potato that had been left on a table in his laboratory.[1] Could each of these droplets represent pure colonies of one species of germs? That observation, and the ability to couple it with an astute question, was a revolutionary step forward in mankind's fight against microbial diseases. As with Koch, research begins with questions whose answers are unknown. The capacity to pose good questions requires an awareness of what is, or might be, relevant, where information is limited and where the knowledge envelope might be pushed forward. Indeed, good clinicians are often well positioned to pose relevant and astute questions. Whatever the source or inspiration, research begins with curiosity.

Creativity: Asking a good question is one thing, but determining how to arrive at a solid answer is quite another. This is where creativity is utterly indispensable. Feeling preoccupied with research—imaging how things work, how to obtain evidence that examines specific hypotheses, anticipating how to overcome obstacles (intellectual, methodological, systemic, and/or financial)—is not so much a hazard of the trade but, rather, a necessity. Despite occasions that may feel onerous, it is the creative process that entices and invigorates researchers most. Although there will always be contingencies that threaten success, imagination usually sets the ceiling on research achievement.

One needs to be creative to devise experimental approaches that are ethical, feasible, rational, and honest. Sometimes, researchers are fortunate enough to be able to rely upon, or adapt, previously proven methods. In other instances, it is far less straightforward. Take, for instance, Thonius Philips van Leeuwenhoek, commonly known as the Father of Microbiology. Sometime in the mid-17th century, this Dutch scientist found himself curious about the nature of things that could not be seen by the human eye. First, however, he needed to perfect the workings of the microscope. With ingenuity, determination, and years of plain hard work, he was finally able to observe and describe—for the first time in recorded history—single-celled organisms, microscopic muscle fibers, bacteria, spermatozoa, and blood flow in capillaries.

Not every methodological challenge is quite as daunting as the one Leeuwenhoek faced, and not every challenge need be faced alone. Modern research and researchers often rely on collaboration. It is important, particularly for novice researchers, to understand that it is perfectly reasonable to look outside of themselves for expertise and the benefits of "collective creativity." Putting together a team (based on trust, along with personal and intellectual compatibility) requires creativity, humility, and good judgment. But whether surrounded by others or isolated within their own thoughts, for researchers, creativity is indispensable.

Cash-In: Conducting research requires the investment of resources, and the "C" for *cash-in* highlights this stage of the research trajectory. *Cash-in* refers to the outlay of intellectual energy, human resources, or money—and in most instances, all three—needed to proceed with launching a study or program of research. Good ideas and even solid, creative methods do not ensure success without some "sweat equity." In this day and age, researchers spend much of their time writing applications, attempting to convince granting agencies their study is worth funding. Although this may not always seem like the most efficient or, dare I say, pleasant way of obtaining research funding, it does ensure that certain principles—such as peer review and a commitment to fairness and excellence—guide whose work is supported.

The need for research funds is by no means a new phenomenon in science. Take the case of Louis Pasteur. Shortly after developing his rabies vaccine, 19 Russian peasants from Smolensk were attacked by a rabid wolf. Upon their arrival in Paris, Pasteur himself provided them treatment, while their countrymen watched and waited. Of the 19, 3 died while the other 16 survived. Pasteur was hailed as a hero. As a show of gratitude, the Tsar of All Russias sent him the cross of Ste. Anne and a hundred thousand francs to start a laboratory, today known as the Institut Pasteur. (We now know that fewer than 1 in 100 people bitten by a rabid animal are likely to get infected, making it easy to speculate that several, if not all, of the deaths among the 19 were as a result of Pasteur's vaccination; www.whale.to/v/pasteur.html.)

Doing research calls for investment. Throughout the ordeal of treating the peasants of Smolensk, Pasteur reportedly could neither eat nor sleep. For most researchers, thoughts regarding study ideas and ways of supporting them—although occasionally disruptive to sleep—are among the first they encounter upon awakening and the last they contemplate before drifting off at night. Although dreams of a benevolent Tsar may be anachronistic, how to sustain one's work is a preoccupation among researchers as old as science itself.

Collection: Having posed the question, devised the methods, and obtained the necessary resources, researchers then move into a collection phase: that is, a time of obtaining whatever information is needed to arrive at some answers. This can be a long and arduous process and requires attention to detail, along with patience and commitment. Take the story of Elie Metchnikoff. Metchnikoff was born in southern Russia in 1845 and is best remembered for his early contributions to human immunity. He was, in fact, awarded the Nobel Prize in 1908 for his novel idea that phagocytes fight off disease by engulfing and destroying harmful bodies such as bacteria. He conducted endless experiments over the course of his career. His dedication, commitment, and willingness to take risks in collecting data knew few bounds.

Using his laboratory workers as human guinea pigs, he would feed them various bacteria to prove their immunity—or not. He himself is said to have swallowed more cholera bacilli than any of them.

In later life, Metchnikoff began to ruminate about aging and death. Turning his scientific energy toward both, he was the first to coin the terms *gerontology* and *thanatology*. Based on fewer facts than inclination, he decided that certain bacilli within the large intestine caused "autointoxication," which he believed could lead to hardening of the arteries and aging. To prove his point, for nearly 20 years, he drank sour milk, which he believed contained Bulgarian bacillus capable of "chasing" wild poisonous bacilli out of the intestine. He continued to test his various juices and excretions until his death at the age of 71.

Collection, that is, the gathering of research data, takes time, attention to detail, and essentially defines the "long haul" of the research process. Although it is rarely glamorous and very few days yield earth-shattering epiphanies, it is the care and integrity that mark this *collection* phase, which determines the solidity of whatever outcome the research might yield.

Cash-Out: As the name implies, *cash-out* is the culmination of the Five Research C's framework. To be explicit, cash-out consists of determining what the research has shown and making those results known. Research describes a process of knowledge generation, and without *cash-out*, for all intents and purposes, there is no new knowledge. The early microbe hunters knew this, and they took the task of *cash-out* seriously. Over the course of nearly 50 years, Anton Van Leeuwenhoek wrote over 500 letters to the Royal Society, reporting until within days of death his studies and observations of various living and nonliving things; "whenever I found out anything remarkable, I have thought it my duty to put down my discovery on paper, so that all ingenious people might be informed thereof." (Leeuwenhoek Letter of June 12, 1716). Robert Koch, the meticulous and stolid German doctor who discovered anthrax bacilli, tuberculous bacilli, and cholera vibrio, presented his initial findings to scientists at the University of Breslau and, later, to the famous Professor Virchow and the Physiological Society at the University of Berlin; his findings rocked the scientific world and paved the way for the future of bacteriology.

Louis Pasteur raised the notion of *cash-out* to an art form. Never one to shy away from attention, each of his discoveries was followed by a wish "to tell the world ... the searcher in him changed into a showman, an exhibitor of stupendous surprises, a missionary in the cause of microbes. The world must know and the people of the world must gasp at this astounding news" (p. 69).

Cashing-out is as critical to research as performance is to music. If profound effort, practice, and creativity amount to little more than silence, the exercise is rather meaningless. Knowledge is meant to be shared, and data that sits idle in a drawer serves no one. Researchers have an obligation to themselves, their colleagues, their funders, and those they study to determine what they have learned, and they must have the courage to follow where

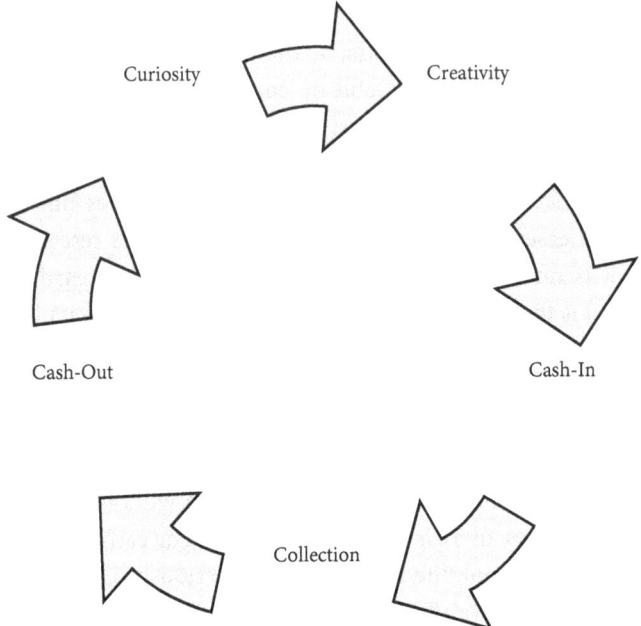

Figure 2.1 The Five Research C's.

their data lead them. They have a similar obligation to make their findings known within a forum—most typically, a peer-reviewed publication—that safeguards integrity and excellence.

A final benefit of *cash-out* is that it perpetuates the research process. Determining what has been learned provides an important opportunity to ask more questions. At the end of a study, researchers are almost always in a strategically better place—in view of what they now know—to reflect on where they need to go next. And so, with curiosity once again aroused, the Five Research C's will have come full circle (Figure 2.1). Once having entered this intriguing, exhilarating, and perpetual cycle of questions and discovery, researchers are rarely, if ever, inclined to take their leave.

Reference

1. de Kruif P. *Microbe Hunters.* Blue Ribbon Books; 1926.

3

Humility and the Practice of Medicine

My relationship with humility has changed over the years. For the longest time, feeling humble was almost entirely about competence and wanting to do right by patients. Humility made me question if I knew enough or was doing enough. Imposter's syndrome and I were well acquainted.

Humility, in healthy doses, can motivate us to reach for whatever high bar we've set for ourselves. Humility is critical in being able to acknowledge what we don't know. (The most dangerous colleagues I've encountered are those who don't know what they don't know.) But like anxiety, too much humility can be paralytic, deflating, like living with a judgmental and punitive taskmaster. While humility didn't have that particular hold on me, there is no doubt it sometimes slowed me down.

But over time, something has changed. Well into what is the third act of my career, I notice humility has become a much easier companion. It has lost its sharp edges and no longer feels unwelcome or hostile. Rather than a harsh voice reminding me of how little I know, or how much more I should be doing, humility's tone seems friendlier, even reassuring. It is now entwined with a wistful awareness that one can never know everything. I find myself reading for the love of learning rather than trying to quell perceived shortcomings. As the years pass, humility concedes that life is fleeting and finite. I will consider myself blessed if time runs out before the waning of curiosity and my sense of wonder.

Humility and the Practice of Medicine. Harvey Max Chochinov. *CMAJ*, 2010;182(11):1217–1218. Reprinted with permission from the publisher.

As Scottish author J.M. Barrie wrote, "Life is a long lesson in humility." At first glance, the topics of medicine and humility would seem an unlikely pairing. After all, training for certainty in the practice of medicine—the slow but steady relinquishment of humility—begins in medical school.

In Search of Dignity. Harvey Max Chochinov, Oxford University Press. © Oxford University Press 2025.
DOI: 10.1093/9780197805145.003.0003

Along the way, ignorance is replaced by knowledge and doubt with assurance. In his book *The Silent World of Doctor and Patient*, Jay Katz[1] states: "Socialization of physicians reinforces the universal human tendency to turn away from uncertainty," letting physicians assume a role as "the bearers of certainty."

But to be humble means to appreciate the limits of your abilities, understanding and importance. For physicians, humility distinguishes between knowing what illness the patient has, and understanding how it feels to have it. Humility differentiates what is clinically indicated from what treatment choices patients deem appropriate; it also separates knowing what *should* happen within specified clinical circumstances from what *does* happen.

Sir William Osler understood that while some things can be known, others must be inferred or experienced. One morning, Osler was discovered by a colleague, "struggling in the effort to pass a stomach tube upon himself, resulting in the ordinary gagging and retching which such a procedure produces in one unaccustomed to it."[2] When asked what he was doing, he replied: "Well, we often pass these on people, and I thought we ought to find out what it feels like ourselves."[2] Wisdom led Osler to appreciate those things that characterize human vulnerability and patienthood; humility helped him understand that there are aspects of human suffering that are not easily penetrable. "This grace of humility," Osler wrote, "is a precious gift."

Years later, Osler protégé Harvey Cushing discovered first-hand the challenges of becoming a patient when he was admitted to hospital for the treatment of severe vascular disease. He bemoaned that "a man deprived of his pants gives up not only independence but identity—even hope."[3] In his cryptic way, Cushing was conceding his humility, by acknowledging that the very essence of who we are and our perceived place in this world is soluble within patienthood. For Cushing, being a patient was a bitter and personal affront. For Osler, it was the cornerstone of compassionate care.

Illness, or even the threat of illness, imposes a state of vulnerability that can undermine a person's sense of self. How physicians *see* patients or, more specifically, how patients perceive themselves to be seen can influence their sense of dignity.[4] We should think of ourselves as mirrors, wherein patients seek some positive reflection or affirmation of themselves. Providing this to patients requires humility. If all we see is the illness, patients may feel that the essence of who they are is being overlooked. If we are distracted, patients may feel unworthy of our attention; if we are too rushed, patients may feel undeserving of our time. And if we deem ourselves more important, patients will feel they are unimportant.

Humility can also facilitate the relinquishment of certainty, which all too often, as Katz writes,[1] serves the purpose of "maintaining professional power and control over the medical decision-making process as well as of maintaining an aura of infallibility." Absolute certainty leaves little room for shared decision-making.

Acknowledging medical uncertainty invites dialogue, providing patients a greater voice in the decision-making process. Physicians who lack humility talk *at* their patients; physicians who are sufficiently humble talk *with* their patients. Talking or partnering with patients can promote empathic connections, which may decrease the risk of physician burnout and enhance the likelihood of job satisfaction.

Like wisdom, humility is not easy to come by. Many patients want to feel that their physician is in control of their disease and have little interest in shared decision-making. Physicians may sense that admitting uncertainty, even to themselves, feels like a breach in their obligation to provide care. Because of the enormous responsibility that comes with the job of doctoring, anxiety is not unusual; admitting one's shortcomings may not salve this anxiety and may even intensify it.[5] Being humble, however, does not mean embracing mediocrity or indecision, any more than clinical confidence need be conflated with arrogance or hubris. And being uncertain does not mean being incompetent. Humility, in fact, is a key driver that commits physicians to the continuous pursuit of knowledge.

Perhaps most humbling of all is accepting that anyone can make a mistake. The emotional toll for physicians involved in medical errors can be profound, and include feelings of guilt, depression, fear, and loss of confidence. While this can happen to any physician, most worrisome are those who don't know what they don't know. Little wonder that competence, as measured by performance on licensure examinations, correlates with a greater likelihood of referring patients for consultation.[6] Clearly, the humility of knowing one's limitations is an important element of competence. This awareness enables physicians to recognize and respect the expertise of others—a cornerstone of gratifying collegial relationships and well-functioning multidisciplinary teams.

The nature of knowledge is impossible to contemplate or grasp in its entirety. In the face of new discoveries and insights, today's medical wisdom may be destined to become yesterday's folly. (The strychnine injections Osler received on his deathbed—at the time a standard practice—are now known to be entirely useless.) The epistemological implications for those who practice medicine are critical. Physicians must be prepared to challenge fundamental assumptions and examine their practice patterns; they must consider credible evidence and be open to change. Humility dictates no matter how great the measure of our reach, we acknowledge the limitations of our grasp.

The truth is everyone, including those we love, confronts health crises; no one is immune. Those of us whose practice can be measured in decades have watched our revered and once powerful mentors grow old and may have helped care for some through their final days of life. Feelings of invincibility are replaced by the realization that patienthood can arrive instantaneously; and that it does not discriminate based on perceived status or power. Indeed, perhaps nothing promotes humility more effectively than the growing realization that little separates us from our patients. Typical of Cushing's experience, the cultivation of humility is often painful and requires a high level of self-awareness and reflective practice.

Within our profession, there is nothing simple about humble pie; but consider taking a bite—it could very well change the way you practise medicine.

Acknowledgements: The author, with all due humility, wishes to thank Dr. Kathleen Foley, for her sage advice, and Prof. Robert Burt, for sharing his wisdom and providing invaluable assistance.

References

1. Katz J. *The Silent World of Doctor and Patient.* Rev. ed. Johns Hopkins University Press; 2002.
2. Bliss M. *William Osler: A Life in Medicine.* Oxford University Press; 1999.
3. Bliss M. *Harvey Cushing: A Life in Surgery.* Oxford University Press; 2005.
4. Chochinov HM. Dignity-conserving care: a new model for palliative care. *JAMA.* 2002;287:2253–2260.
5. Burt R. Doctors vs. lawyers: the perils of perfectionism. *St Louis Univ Law J.* 2009;53:1177–1188.
6. Tamblyn R, Laprise R, Hanley JA, et al. Adverse events associated with prescription drug cost-sharing among poor and elderly persons. *JAMA.* 2001; 285:421–429.

4

Thinking Outside the Box

Depression, Hope, and Meaning at the End of Life

Anyone practicing medicine long enough recalls patients who leave an indelible mark. "Jacques," whose story I recount in this article, was one such patient. He taught me a lot about personhood, the importance of affirming someone's ongoing value, and how precious human connections really are. Despite a gratifying career in music, which saw him collect friends and lovers in various "ports around the world" (as he described it), Jacques never committed himself to a life partner, nor did he have a family of his own. For Jacques, being a musician had always felt like enough—that is, until he found himself facing advanced, life-threatening cancer. I recall him once lamenting there was no one in the waiting room, nor anyone anxiously anticipating his arrival home, to ask how his appointment had gone.

I wrote this article about "thinking outside the box" when I realized my professional training hadn't prepared me for a holistic perspective and the likes of Jacques. He taught me that to appreciate suffering, one must try to grasp the entirety of a patient's experience, rather than somehow forcing that experience into a reductive or restrictive framework. It would have been much easier to formulate my understanding of Jacques as a senior gentleman with a major depression, emerging in the course of a terminal illness, and to prescribe and monitor medications accordingly. While that would have been simpler, it would not have been sufficient. What Jacques yearned for and needed was to be seen, to be heard, to be appreciated as someone with an abiding artistic spirit, which, to the very end, not even cancer could claim.

Shortly before he died, Jacques gave me a cassette recording of one of his final performances. To this day I keep it in the drawer of my bedside night table. There are some things you can never part with.

In Search of Dignity. Harvey Max Chochinov, Oxford University Press. © Oxford University Press 2025.
DOI: 10.1093/9780197805145.003.0004

Thinking Outside the Box: Depression, Hope, and Meaning at the End of Life. Harvey Max Chochinov. *Journal of Palliative Medicine*, 2003;6(6):973–977. Reprinted with permission from Mary Ann Liebert, Inc. publishers.

Introduction

I met Jacques 3 years prior to his death (Jacques was not his real name, but I think the panache and elegance of this alias would have pleased and suited him perfectly). His head-and-neck surgeon had referred him to me for a psychiatric consultation, 6 months after a base tongue resection and left neck dissection because of squamous cell carcinoma. The consultation request contained descriptors such as depressive symptoms, sleep disturbance, and a general request for further follow-up and treatment; for all intents and purposes, a typical—even generic—consultation request for someone in my line of work.

The surgeon's note covertly suggested that there were several key issues needing to be addressed. Was Jacques clinically depressed? Did his symptoms imply the presence of a psychiatric syndrome? Would diagnosis lead to the recommendation of a specific treatment? Cause, effect, response, and outcome: all reasonable questions within the context of a contemporary medical, psychiatric model. In this case, cause being the assault of a life-threatening, disfiguring cancer; effect being a likely diagnosis of a clinical depression; response, the possible prescription of a well-chosen psychopharmaceutical; and outcome, the hope or wish that Jacques would be able to carry on, or at the very least, face his future with some degree of equanimity or hope.

This model or paradigm has obvious merits and has benefited multitudes of patients. In contemporary psychiatric practice, the Diagnostic and Statistical Manual of Mental Disorders, currently in its fourth edition (DSM-IV), has had a tremendous impact on patient care and our ability to describe human behavior.[1] It has also deeply affected, for better and worse, those practitioners who apply it. Models, like boxes, provide a neat and readily available place to put things. Eliciting descriptions of symptoms, accurate diagnostic labeling, and targeted therapeutic interventions can each serve the cause of promoting quality patient care. There is, however, a comfort level in being able to categorize, label, pigeonhole—file and save—that can sometimes contaminate or even supersede the often more nebulous task of coming to a real appreciation of the patient's inner experience.

Looking Beyond Depression

Understanding Jacques' inner life, and a sense of the complexity of that inner life, extended far beyond the question of whether he was depressed. During the time I knew him, there were indeed periods when he seemed to benefit somewhat from the antidepressant trials I initiated; in response to a pervasive depressed mood, occasional feelings of hopelessness, loss of interest or pleasure in most things, and feelings of guilt over perceived past indiscretions, it seemed a reasonable therapeutic maneuver.

Palliative care researchers have tried to sensitize the field regarding the importance of understanding psychiatric morbidity that can arise among patients with life-limiting diseases.[2-7] The past decade has seen studies that have examined how to apply standard diagnostic approaches for depression among dying patients, prevalence studies of psychiatric disorders in this vulnerable patient population, brief screening approaches to help clinicians identify depressive syndromes in palliative care settings, and relatively few interventional studies looking at psychopharmaceutical and psychotherapeutic applications for depressed patients nearing death.

The source of Jacques' angst, however, was far more difficult to influence, compared to the task of adjusting his doses of Paxil, or closer to dying, methylphenidate. Until his cancer diagnosis at the age of 72, Jacques had been a professional classical violist. Music had been the center of his life, and the viola, his only chosen life partner. His career had seen him play with all the great orchestras of the world and befriend many of the world's finest musicians. One would describe him, as I recall the cover photograph from his last CD, as suave and dashing; a full head of dark hair combed straight back, clean-shaven, black tuxedo and white cravat, cradling his beloved viola, his gaze cast forward.

His illness sequelae included some mild facial disfigurement, a long and hard struggle to learn to manage his own secretions, and total reliance on enteral tube feedings for the remainder of his days. These bodily assaults paled in comparison to the assault on his core sense of self or spirit. His cancer surgery involved the resection of the left base of his tongue, removal of the adjacent neck strap musculature and spinal accessory nerve, and a radical forearm free flap from his nondominant hand to reconstruct the surgical deficient. Although right-handed, his left hand—the hand he used to finger the world's complete repertoire for the viola—soon developed loss of dexterity caused by forearm strictures, making him no longer able to play music.

The session in which we discussed his decision to send his viola out of province for safekeeping had the quality of planning a funeral for one's only true love. I recall him saying, "My doctor tells me my prognosis is good for the future. What future?" Up until the end, he teetered between contemplating suicide (while never taking any measures to hasten his death) and trying to hold on to the remnants of those few things that still mattered.

Stepping Outside of the Box

The euthanasia and assisted suicide debate has unwittingly moved forward some areas of psychiatric palliative care research. Trying to understand why some patients might lose the wish to go on living has seen researchers extend beyond the conventional DSM-IV paradigm and look at sources of distress that have informed the field of palliative care.[8-11] Several independent groups, for example, have confirmed the dominance of depression as a predictor of desire for death, or interest in physician-assisted suicide.[8,12,13] Those same investigators have also looked at the construct of hopelessness and found it to be an ardent predictor of a wish to die, even among patients close to death.[8,14,15] Dr. Ben Zylicz of The Netherlands argues that in a country where euthanasia and assisted suicide are legal, exemplary palliative care is particularly important in staving off hopelessness and the wish to end one's life.[16]

Within jurisdictions where death-hastening measures are legal, researchers have helped us understand the various factors that can move patients toward life-terminating measures.[17-23] As one might expect, depression and pain figure prominently, but constructs such as being a burden to others, loss of sense of purpose, meaning, and hope, and notably loss of dignity all emerge as significant forces that can move patients toward a hastened death. Clearly, an honest engagement of these issues requires that palliative care clinicians and researchers conceive of ways to expand, if not step well outside of a too-narrowly defined model of end-of-life care.

The need for a broad and inclusive model of palliative care is further supported by the observation that symptoms relating to psychological distress and existential concerns are even more prevalent than pain and other physical symptoms among those with life-limiting conditions.[24] The Institute of Medicine recently released a report entitled, *Approaching*

Death: Improving Care at the End of Life.[25] The domains of quality supportive care they identified from a professional perspective include: (1) overall quality of life; (2) physical well-being and functioning; (3) psychosocial well-being and functioning; (4) spiritual well-being; (5) patient perception of care; and (6) family well-being and functioning.[18] Singer and colleagues[26] reported the domains of supportive care that were found to be most important from the perspective of cancer patients include: (1) receiving adequate pain and symptom control; (2) avoiding inappropriate prolongation of dying; (3) achieving a sense of spiritual peace; (4) relieving burden; and (5) strengthening relationships with loved ones. Moadel and colleagues[27] surveyed 248 patients with cancer and asked them what their most important needs were. Nearly half indicated they needed help overcoming fears, finding hope, meaning in life; finding peace of mind and finding spiritual resources.[27]

A national survey by Meier and colleagues[22] found that "loss of meaning in life" was a reason highly cited by physicians as to why patients request assisted suicide. Clearly, from the vantage point of professionals and patients alike, acknowledging and addressing issues such as meaning, purpose, and hope needs to be included within the realm of quality end-of-life care.

New Boxes

Broadening the paradigm, expanding the model, finding new boxes, call it what you will, but within palliative medicine, there is evidence that this has started to happen. For example, Kissane and colleagues[27] have proposed "demoralization syndrome" as a diagnostic entity within palliative care, with hopelessness, loss of meaning, and existential distress identified as its core features. They suggest that this syndrome can be differentiated from depression, and is associated with chronic medical illness, disability, bodily disfigurement, fear of loss of dignity, social isolation, and—where there is a subjective sense of incompetence—feelings of greater dependency on others or the perception of being a burden. Because of the sense of impotence or helplessness, those with the syndrome are thought to have a propensity to progress toward a desire to die or commit suicide.

Over the last 5 years, our group has been studying the construct of dying with dignity, in an attempt to understand what supports, or conversely, what undermines the dignity of a patient nearing death.[29-31] These studies led to the development of a model of dignity in the terminally ill, which incorporates physical, psychological, and spiritual, and social aspects of the illness experience (illness related concerns, dignity conserving repertoire, and social dignity inventory, respectively). Each of these broad categories contains subthemes that further elucidate components of a broadly based, empirically validated dignity-conserving model of end-of-life care. Besides including issues pertaining to hope, meaning, and purpose, the model suggests that dignity concerns can be multifactorial. For example, for some patients, a sense that nothing of one's life will be transcendent of death—a concept we labeled generativity and legacy—was experienced as an assault on dignity. For many patients, maintaining dignity was highly dependent on how they perceived themselves to be seen. Therefore, supporting the perception that patients maintain their sense of worth, as affirmed by those who care for them, is a powerful dignity-conserving strategy.

The Dignity Model in the Terminally Ill also provides the theoretical foundation for a novel, brief, individual intervention we have coined Dignity Therapy.[30] Dignity Therapy is currently the focus of an international feasibility study, being piloted with palliative care patients in Winnipeg, Canada, and Perth, Australia. This intervention incorporates those facets from the model that are most likely to bolster the dying patients' sense of worth, purpose, or meaning. Patients are offered the opportunity to speak to issues they hold to be most important, such as recounting aspects of their life they feel proudest of, things they feel are or were most meaningful, the personal history they would most want remembered; or words they might provide in the service of helping to look after their family and friends, such as hopes, wishes, or directions for those they will soon leave behind. Because of the importance of generativity as a significant dignity theme, Dignity Therapy sessions are taped, transcribed, edited for clarity, and quickly returned to the patient. The creation of a tangible product that will live beyond the patient acknowledges the importance of generativity as a salient dignity issue. The immediacy of the returned transcript is intended to bolster the patient's sense of purpose, meaning, and worth, while tangibly experiencing their thoughts and words as continuing to be valued. If shown to be effective, this will be one of the few new non-pharmacologic interventions for suffering or psychosocial distress that so often arises among dying patients.

Meaning-Centered Group Psychotherapy

The work of Dr. William Breitbart has been seminal in the field of psycho-oncology and palliative care.[3,4,13,15,32,33] The studies published by his team have provided crucial descriptive data regarding the nature of depression, delirium, pain, and other various sources of symptom distress commonly seen in patients with life-limiting conditions. What is perhaps most notable about his recent work featured in this issue of *Innovations*,[34] is the evolution toward interventional studies targeted at enhancing spiritual well-being among patients with advanced cancer.[35,36] The novel intervention they have coined meaning-centered group psychotherapy is based on the concepts and principles of Viktor Frankl's logotherapy.[37] Frankl's work raised awareness regarding spiritual issues and the importance of meaning or the *will to meaning* as a driving force or instinct in human experience.

Frankl's logotherapy was not designed for the treatment of those with a life-threatening illness. Nevertheless, Breitbart and colleagues[34] have incorporated these concepts of meaning and spirituality into their psychotherapeutic work with advanced cancer patients, many of whom seek guidance and help in dealing with issues of sustaining meaning, hope, and understanding impending death in the context of their lives. Clearly, meaning-centered therapies are not a panacea for all sources of suffering, nor are they likely to be applied effectively to everyone. Patients will vary in the degree to which they experience angst in terms of lost meaning and hope, and enthusiasm for new approaches should not distract us from paying close attention to depressive disorders and cognitive limitations (including pseudodementia). In some instances, these conditions may render meaning-centered approaches ineffective, while in others they may be applied as an adjunct to more conventional psychiatry interventions. That having been said, the incorporation of interventions such as these will not only address a vital therapeutic need but will broaden the model of palliative medicine that will enable it to provide dignity-conserving care for patients—and their families—facing death.

Conclusions

I last saw Jacques a few days before he died. He was in the hospital at the time, vaguely confused but nevertheless aware of who I was and that I sensed his recent, grave deterioration in health. During our last visit, I was thinking about the notion of Jacques' dignity, and the extent to which preconceived models or boxes had failed to encapsulate the full extent of his suffering. I recall the presence of a nurse at the foot of his bed, attending to charting or some such mechanical task. Turning to her, I said, "Did you know that Jacques was a professional musician? He played viola with all the world's finest orchestras and musicians, including the likes of Leonard Bernstein, Herbert Von Karajan, Jean-Pierre Rampal, Vladimir Ashkenazy, and Glenn Gould." (I must admit, those that I could not remember I simply made up.) The effect was immediate and, I thought, profound. Jacques broke out in a full body blush, and a smile his face could barely contain. Later that morning, I overheard his nurse sharing the impressive details of Jacques' glorious past with one of her colleagues. He was no longer simply an elderly male with an oral malignancy and secondary complications, admitted for palliative care, but someone deserved of honor, respect, and esteem—words corresponding to the definition of dignity itself.

Not every patient necessarily has an account of former glory. Yet every patient, without exception, has a past, a story—something that ultimately and uniquely defines who and what they were or continue to be. Dignity-conserving care, in part, is comprised of being able to identify and acknowledge those fundamental and defining aspects of personhood. Seeing patients for who and what they are or were, profoundly enhances their quality of end-of-life care. This will require care staff to be trained and sensitized to appreciate the importance of their own perceptions toward patients for whom they care. Helping patients to find a sense of purpose, meaning, and dignity requires us to step outside of the box and develop a model of palliation that incorporates patient experience in its entirety. By so doing, palliative medicine stands to accomplish so much more, and patients nearing the end of life deserve nothing less.

References

1. American Psychiatric Association. *Diagnostic and Statistical Manual of Mental Disorders.* 4th ed. American Psychiatric Association; 1994.
2. Chochinov HM, Wilson, KG, Enns M, Lander S. The prevalence of depression in the terminally ill: effects of diagnostic criteria and symptom threshold judgments. *Am J Psychiatry.* 1994;151:537–540.
3. Breitbart W, Bruera E, Chochinov HM, Lynch M. Neuropsychiatric syndromes and psychological symptoms in patients with advanced cancer. *J Pain Symptom Manage.* 1995;10:131–141.

4. Breitbart W, Chochinov HM, Passik S. Psychiatric aspects of palliative care. In: Doyle D, Hanks GWC, MacDonald N, eds. *Oxford Textbook of Palliative Medicine*. 2nd ed. Oxford University Press; 1998:933–954.

5. Holland JC. Improving the human side of cancer care: psycho-oncology's contribution. *Cancer J*. 2001;7:458–471.

6. Chochinov HM, Wilson K, Enns M, Lander S. Are you depressed? Screening for depression in the terminally ill. *Am J Psychiatry*. 1997;154:674–676.

7. Chochinov HM. Psychiatry and the terminally ill. *Can J Psychiatry*. 2000;45:143–150.

8. Wilson KG, Scott JF, Graham ID, et al. Attitudes of terminally ill patients toward euthanasia and physician-assisted suicide. *Arch Intern Med*. 2000;160:2454–2460.

9. Block SD. Perspectives on care at the close of life. Psychological considerations, growth, and transcendence at the end of life: the art of the possible. *JAMA*. 2001;285:2898–2905.

10. McPhee SJ, Markowitz AJ. Psychological considerations, growth, and transcendence at the end of life: the art of the possible. *JAMA*. 2001;286:3002.

11. Lo B, Ruston D, Kates LW, et al. Discussing religious and spiritual issues at the end of life: a practical guide for physicians. *JAMA*. 2002;287:749–754.

12. Chochinov HM, Wilson KG, Enns M, et al. Desire for death in the terminally ill. *Am J Psychiatry*. 1995;152:1185–1191.

13. Breitbart W, Rosenfeld BD, Passik SD. Interest in physician-assisted suicide among ambulatory HIV-infected patients. *Am J Psychiatry*. 1996;153:238–242.

14. Chochinov HM, Wilson KG, Enns M, Lander S. Depression, hopelessness, and suicidal ideation in the terminally ill. *Psychosomatics*. 1998;39:366–370.

15. Breitbart W, Rosenfeld B, Pessin H. Depression, hopelessness, and desire for hastened death in terminally ill patients with cancer. *JAMA*. 2000;284:2907–2911.

16. Zylicz B. Palliative care and euthanasia in The Netherlands: observations of a Dutch physician. In: Foley K, Hendin H, eds. *The Case Against Assisted Suicide: For the Right to End-of-Life Care*. Johns Hopkins University Press; 2002:122–143.

17. van der Maas PJ, Van Delden JJM, Pijnenborg L, Looman CWN. Euthanasia and other medical decisions concerning the end of life. *Lancet*. 1991;338:669–674.

18. van der Maas PJ, van der Wal G, Haverkate I. Euthanasia, physician-assisted suicide, and other medical practices involving the end of life in the Netherlands, 1990–1995. *N Engl J Med*. 1996;335:1699–1705.

19. Back AL, Wallace JI, Starks HE, Pearlman RA. Physician-assisted suicide and euthanasia in Washington state: patient requests and physician responses. *JAMA*. 1996;275:919–925.

20. Emanuel EJ, Fairclough DL, Daniels ER, Clarridge BR. Euthanasia and physician-assisted suicide: attitudes and experiences of oncology patients, oncologists, and the public. *Lancet*. 1996;347:1805–1810.

21. Ganzini L, Nelson HD, Schmidt TA, et al. Physicians' experiences with the Oregon Death with Dignity Act. *N Engl J Med*. 2000;342:557–563.

22. Meier DE, Emmons CA, Wallenstein S, et al. A national survey of physician-assisted suicide and euthanasia in the United States. *N Engl J Med*. 1998;338:1193–1201.

23. Sullivan AD, Hedberg K, Fleming DW. Legalized physician-assisted suicide in Oregon—the second year. *N Engl J Med*. 2000;342:598–604.

24. Portenoy RK, Thaler HT, Kornblith AB, et al. Symptom prevalence, characteristics and distress in a cancer population. *Qual Life Res*. 1994;3:183–189.

25. Field MJ, Cassel CK, eds. *Approaching Death: Improving Care at the End of Life*. National Academy Press; 1997.

26. Singer PA, Martin DK, Kelner M. Quality end-of-life care: patients' perspectives. *JAMA*. 1999;281:163–168.

27. Moadel A, Morgan C, Fatone A. Seeking meaning and hope: self-reported spiritual and existential needs among an ethnically-diverse cancer patient population. *Psychooncology*. 1999;8:378–385.

28. Kissane DW, Clarke DM, Street AF. Demoralization syndrome—a relevant psychiatric diagnosis for palliative care. *J Palliat Care.* 2001;17:12–21.

29. Chochinov HM, Hack T, McClement S, et al. Dignity in the terminally ill: an empirical model. *Soc Sci Med.* 2002;54:433–443.

30. Chochinov HM. Dignity-conserving care: a new model for palliative care. *JAMA.* 2002;287:2253–2260.

31. Chochinov HM, Hack T, Hassard T, et al. Dignity in the terminally ill. *Lancet.* 2002;360:2026–2030.

32. Breitbart W, Kaim M, Rosenfeld B. Clinicians' perceptions of barriers to pain management in AIDS. *J Pain Symptom Manage.* 1999;18:203–212.

33. Breitbart W, Gibson C, Tremblay A. The delirium experience: delirium recall and delirium-related distress in hospitalized patients with cancer, their spouses/caregivers, and their nurses. *Psychosomatics.* 2002;43:183–194.

34. Breitbart W, Heller KS. Reframing hope: meaning-centered care for patients near the end of life. *J Palliat Med.* 2003;6:979–988.

35. Breitbart W. Spirituality and meaning in supportive care: spirituality- and meaning-centered group psychotherapy interventions in advanced cancer. *Support Care Cancer.* 2002;10:272–280.

36. Greenstein M, Breitbart W. Cancer and the experience of meaning: a group psychotherapy program for people with cancer. *Am J Psychother.* 2000;54:486–500.

37. Frankl VF. *Man's Search for Meaning.* 4th ed. Beacon Press; 1959/1992.

SECTION 2

DIGNITY . . . AND MORE DIGNITY

5

Dignity and the Eye of the Beholder

While the article by Dr. James Brown was pivotal in launching my research career, the paper by Dr. Paul Van Der Maas turned my attention toward dignity. He discovered that loss of dignity was the most common reason, according to Dutch physicians, their patients sought out euthanasia or assisted suicide. This was the first time it occurred to me this was something that needed to be examined. If dignity was worth dying for, dignity was worth studying.

Any serious research endeavor begins with examining the literature. This search revealed that dignity was a frequently cited, albeit nebulous, contentious, and politicized, term. For those who supported physician-hastened death, the argument of autonomy—my body, my choice—was ultimately framed as a matter of dignity. The opposing argument held that the taking of human life, the violation of the Hippocratic Oath, was an assault on human dignity. As researchers, our position was to step away from any political or ideological stance and, for the first time, to ask patients nearing death to help us understand the importance of dignity.

Our various studies on dignity and the detailed findings are now well embedded in the palliative care literature. This article, "Dignity and the Eye of the Beholder," summarizes some key early insights, along with what I consider my first "dignity epiphany." I had always thought good palliative care—which focuses intently on optimizing quality of life—was achieved by what one did to or with patients. Yet our data revealed that the most significant factor that determined patient dignity was how they perceived themselves to be seen by their healthcare provider. In other words, how we see our patient—how we perceive and appreciate them—fundamentally shapes every clinical encounter and overall patient experience. This applies not only within the realm of palliative care, but across all of medicine.

This epiphany led to other studies and further contemplation of what shapes the healthcare provider's gaze, and how bias can influence and sometimes taint our clinical impressions. Acknowledging patients as whole persons ensures they are genuinely seen and known above and beyond

In Search of Dignity. Harvey Max Chochinov, Oxford University Press. © Oxford University Press 2025.
DOI: 10.1093/9780197805145.003.0005

whatever ailment they have. It also ensures alignment between how we see them and how they see themselves. At its core, Dignity Therapy requires finding out who the patient is and how they would want to be remembered.

This article recalls Mr. J, the first patient to participate in Dignity Therapy. He left an indelible mark on my professional life and research. When I was asked to see him in consultation, he did not have any psychiatric disorder that I could discern. I decided to offer him a prototype of Dignity Therapy (at that time, we were still working out the details). I remember explaining how I imagined it would work, anticipating the things we might talk about, and how that would evolve into a generativity document. There was no arm twisting; he was immediately interested and wanted to take part.

I remember the last time I saw Mr. J, he was too sick and weak to take the document from my hand. His wife, who was sitting at his bedside, received the document, and said, "This will be a blessing to our family." I hope it was. Mr. J certainly was a blessing in my life and work, and helped move the field of palliative care in a direction that has embraced broader considerations of human dignity.

Dignity and the Eye of the Beholder. Harvey Max Chochinov. *Journal of Clinical Oncology.* 2004;22(7):1336–1340. Reprinted with permission from the publisher.

Mr. J was a 67-year-old man with an end-stage gastrointestinal malignancy. Having decided he no longer wished to go on living, he had gone on a hunger strike, precipitating an admission to an inpatient tertiary palliative care unit. He reported that, aside from some minor discomforts, his symptom management was quite reasonable. Psychiatric consultation was initiated to determine if depression might be a factor influencing his wish to die. While he was not overtly suicidal, and in fact seemed ambivalent about his wish to die, he did state, "if I were in a European country where I could 'press the button now,' I would." After careful evaluation, it was determined that rather than depression, the driving force behind his desire for death was a sense that life no longer had meaning, purpose, nor hope. While he spoke of a lingering wish to participate in various life activities, he bemoaned the fact that his body was simply too weak and too ill to allow him to do so. That being the case, he expressed the conviction that breathing had become redundant, his life had no worth, and there was little reason for him to carry on.

How can we offer comfort to patients whose distress is primarily in the realm of the existential, or beyond the reach of an easily administered psychopharmaceutical or analgesic drug? While these matters are often deferred to the expertise of pastoral care professionals, there is a growing movement—particularly in reference to dying patients—for physicians to expand their caring with attentiveness to psychosocial, existential, or spiritual suffering.[1-3] In the absence of a clinical depression or formal psychiatric disorder, the paucity of therapeutic options or formatted approaches can leave oncology practitioners at somewhat of a loss. There may be aspects of despair toward the end of life that may be inherent to the dying process itself. If such distress is not primarily an aberration of neurochemistry, but rather reflects a paucity of hope, meaning, and self-worth, what can be done to safeguard or enhance those life-sustaining attributes? And if loss of meaning, hope, and self-worth are the essence of such despair, what implications does this have for palliative care providers?

The Wish to Die

The expression of a desire for death, or of a loss of will to live, is often misconstrued as being synonymous with a request for euthanasia or assisted suicide. There is good evidence, however, that in the context of advanced illness, desire for death can be thought of along a continuum. At its most extreme, desire for death is synonymous with suicidal intent and preoccupation with the wish to die. Far more common, however, are the many patients who, over the course of their cancer illness, experience occasional and fleeting thoughts that not waking up to another day might offer the kind of escape and comfort they perceive life can no longer provide.[4,5] People tire of pain, disability, changing roles, mounting losses, and fewer prospects for remediation. In the face of depression, poor symptom control, and lack of appropriate supports, these thoughts can become overwhelming. Conversely, in response to appropriate palliation and the rallying of a community of support, thoughts about the wish to die can dramatically recede.[4-10]

A variety of studies over the last decade have attempted to profile those patients whose distress has led to a request for hastened death.[4-9,11,12] The social policy implications of these studies aside, the implications for practitioners attempting to provide quality end-of-life care are substantial. This literature has provided clear evidence that patients expressing a consistent wish to die are most often burdened by various physical symptoms (particularly pain, dyspnea, and fatigue), psychological symptoms (especially depression), lack of social support, along with various existential concerns (especially worries about being a burden to others), losing control, hopelessness, and general concern that the future only holds a worsening of their distress.

But what does it mean to be hopeless in the face of a hopeless prognosis? Several studies have reported that hopelessness is an ardent predictor of suicidal ideation, even among the terminally ill, and that hopelessness is usually most pronounced in patients meeting criteria for major depression.[13-15] While depression is present in a minority of dying patients (10% to 25%, depending on what criteria are used and the way they are applied), neither hopelessness nor depression define the experience of most individuals nearing death.[16] If hopelessness is not based on prognostic expectation, how is it then to be understood?

Dignity in the Terminally Ill

To broach the question of hope in patients with advanced illness, we must look toward the broader notion of what it means to die with dignity. Several studies have drawn a connection between loss of dignity toward the end of life and a wish to die. Some Dutch studies have reported that loss of dignity, according to physicians, is the most highly cited reason why patients seek out and receive assistance hastening their death.[11] The topic of dignity, however, has not been extensively researched, and most often enters palliative care discourse within the context of social policy and philosophical or religious considerations. Thus, while many caregivers give lip service to the idea of providing care that preserves dignity at the end of life, few specifically target maintaining dignity as an objective standard of quality end-of-life care.

Over the last 5 years, some of the first studies have been published regarding the issue of dignity among the dying.[17-19] One such study examined a cohort of 213 terminal cancer patients, with a life expectancy of less than 6 months, asking them to rate their sense of dignity.[17] Of these patients, only 16 patients (7.5%) indicated that loss of dignity was a significant concern. These patients were far more likely to have significantly increased pain, decreased quality of life, difficulty with bowel functioning, heightened dependency needs (bathing, dressing, incontinence), loss of will to live, increased desire for death, depression, hopelessness, and anxiety. This report also noted that the issue of appearance seemed to highly correlate with perceptions of personal dignity. For those near the end of life, the notion of appearance extended beyond mere looks, and included their own perception of how they are seen by others.

Mr. J, being a man with an end-stage bowel malignancy, had many of the various medical problems that go along with this diagnosis. However, to have known him only in this capacity would have overlooked his core identity and placed his sense of dignity in jeopardy. If care provider perception is limited to gastrointestinal considerations, then the patient's accurate perception of how he is perceived is as an advanced bowel cancer. Therefore, appreciation and acknowledgment of his core identity as a father, grandfather, husband, and someone with a diverse range of interests, can alter the perception of those looking after Mr. J, offering him the comfort of knowing that personhood has been acknowledged and affirmed.

The Dignity Model

An empirically based model of dignity in the terminally ill has been developed (Figure 5.1).[18,19] This model provides caregivers a therapeutic map, incorporating a broad range of physical, psychological, social, and existential

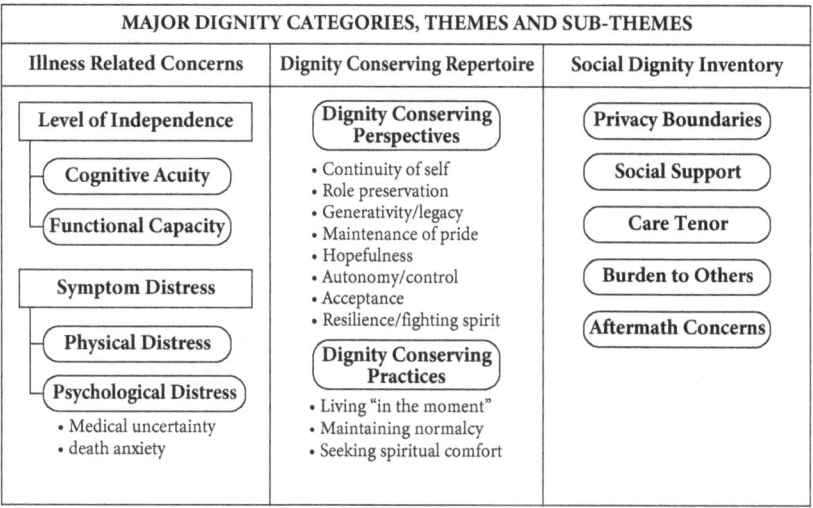

Figure 5.1 Reprinted with permission from Social Science and Medicine, Vol 54, No 3, pp 433–443, Chochinov et al: "Dignity in the terminally ill: An empirical model." Copyright 2002, with permission from Elsevier.

issues that may affect individual perceptions of dignity. While many pallia-tive care clinicians provide empathic care, the Dignity Model offers a broad framework that can be used to inform dignity-conserving care.

Three major categories have emerged from qualitative analysis of dying patients' perceptions of their sense of dignity,[18,19] including: (1) Illness-Related Issues; (2) Dignity Conserving Repertoire; and (3) Social Dignity Inventory. These categories refer to broad issues that determine how individuals experience a sense of dignity during their approaching death. Each of these categories contains several carefully defined themes and sub-themes, serving as the foundation for a model of understanding dignity amongst the dying.

Illness-Related Issues and Concerns

These are issues that derive from the illness itself and threaten to or impinge on the patient's sense of dignity. The defining characteristic of these issues is that they are illness mediated, and very specific to the patient's illness experi-ence. The two broad themes subsumed within this category consist of "Level of Independence" (which is determined by one's ability to maintain cogni-tive acuity, as well as functional capacity, referring to the ability to perform daily living tasks), and "Symptom Distress." Symptom distress was further divided into the subthemes of physical distress and psychological distress. Psychological distress was divided into the following sub-themes: (1) un-certainty (i.e., the distress associated with the uncertainties of one's health status) and (2) death anxiety (i.e., worry or fear specifically associated with the process or anticipation of death and dying).

Dignity Conserving Repertoire

The second major category that emerged was the Dignity Conserving Repertoire. This category was divided into two major themes, including Dignity Conserving Perspectives and Dignity Conserving Practices.

Dignity Conserving Perspectives are internally held qualities, or a world view consisting of eight sub-themes, including (1) continuity of self (a sense that the essence of who one is continues to remain intact, despite one's advancing illness), (2) role preservation (the ability to continue to function in usual roles, as a way of maintaining a sense congruence with prior views of self), (3) generativity/legacy (the solace and comfort in knowing that something lasting of oneself will transcend death), (4) maintaining pride (the ability to maintain a positive sense of self regard or respect), (5) maintaining hope (an ability to see life as enduring, or having sustained meaning or purpose), (6) autonomy/control (a sense of control over one's life circumstances), (7) acceptance (the internal process of resigning one's self to changing life circumstances), and (8) resilience/fighting spirit (the mental determination to overcome illness-related concerns and optimize quality of life).

Dignity Conserving Practices refer to a variety of personal approaches or techniques that patients use to bolster or maintain their sense of dignity. Three components of these practices were identified: "Living in the Moment" (focusing on immediate issues or tasks in the service of not worrying about the future), "Maintaining Normalcy" (continuous or routine behaviors, which help individuals manage day-to-day challenges), and "Seeking Spiritual Comfort" (turning toward or finding solace in one's religious or spiritual belief system).

Social Dignity Inventory

This refers to the quality of interactions with others that enhance or detract from one's sense of dignity. The defining characteristic of this inventory is that it refers to external sources or issues that nevertheless impinge on a patient's sense of dignity. Five primary inventory themes were identified, including: (1) Privacy Boundaries (the extent to which one's personal environment is encroached on while receiving care or support), (2) Social Support (the presence of an available and helpful community of friends, family, or health care providers), (3) Care Tenor (the attitude others demonstrate when interacting with the patient that may or may not promote dignity), (4) Burden to Others (the distress engendered by having to rely on others for various aspects of one's personal care or management), and (5) Aftermath Concerns (the worry or fears in anticipation of the burden or challenges that one's death will impose on others).

This Dignity Model provides an empirically derived framework, helping us understand the notion of dignity in those nearing death. Furthermore, it provides a foundation on which to both understand how a dying patient may experience a waning of their dignity, and, in turn, provides direction for how to construct dignity-enhancing interventions for patients nearing death. One such intervention, for example, is a brief psychotherapeutic intervention called Dignity Therapy. This approach comprises tape-recorded sessions, which gives patients the opportunity to speak to aspects of life of which they feel proudest, things that are, or were, most meaningful, and their personal history they would most want remembered. They are also able to speak about what they might provide in the service of helping to look after their soon-to-be bereft loved ones (Table 1). These sessions are transcribed, edited, and returned to the patient, thereby bolstering the patient's sense of purpose, meaning, and worth, while tangibly experiencing their thoughts and words as having continued value, and satisfying their generativity needs.

Mr. J was invited to participate in the Dignity Therapy clinical trial. From the moment he agreed to do so, he indicated that he would defer any decision to "push the button, at least not until this task was completed." He used this therapeutic trial, mere days before his natural death, as an opportunity to share recollections about his own parents; the trials of living through a devastating war; life as an immigrant; getting married and developing a vocation; the deep and tragic losses that continued to weigh heavily; and the joyful pride he took in his children, grandchildren, and extended community. The

Table 1 Dignity Psychotherapy Question Protocol

Tell me a little about your life history; particularly the parts that you either remember most, or think are the most important? When did you feel most alive?

Are there specific things that you would want your family to know about you, and are there particular things you would want them to remember?

What are the most important roles you have played in life (family roles, vocational roles, community service roles, etc)? Why were they so important to you, and what do you think you accomplished in those roles?

What are your most important accomplishments, and what do you feel most proud of?

Are there particular things that you feel still need to be said to your loved ones, or things that you would want to take the time to say once again? What are your hopes and dreams for your loved ones?

What have you learned about life that you would want to pass along to others? What advice or words of guidance would you wish to pass along to your (son, daughter, husband, wife, parents, other(s))?

Are there words or perhaps even instructions you would like to offer your family, to help prepare them for the future?

In creating this permanent record, are there other things that you would like included?

---

role of the therapist was to gently facilitate these poignant disclosures, and to convey the message that Mr. J's words, thoughts, and feelings were important, and that the task of sharing these disclosures was profoundly meaningful.

In the absence of such a trial, how might a healthcare provider otherwise attend to Mr. J's distress? While his suffering is considerable, it does not appear to solicit a specific medical response. Intuitively, what might be done? Likely, little time would pass before a care provider would take a seat at the bedside and begin to talk, or perhaps simply listen. And what might be said or heard? The first words would likely be questions about what is happening to him, what matters to him, how he understands what is taking place. Perhaps the care provider might find himself or herself listening to some personal or intimate thought or reflection. In either case, the provider's presence holds tremendous therapeutic potency; by taking a place at the bedside, whether asking questions about what matters, or listening to heartfelt disclosures, the provider becomes the beholder. By listening to patients, our perception of who they are extends beyond the confines of their illness, thereby shifting the patient's perception of how they are seen and heard. Validation of their concerns and ascribing meaning to their experience, according to the Dignity Model, can bolster hope, even for those whose illness has long since extended beyond the reach of cure. The reflection that patients see of themselves in the eye of the care provider must ultimately affirm their sense of dignity. At least in part, it would appear, dignity resides in the eye of the beholder.

References

1. Thiel MM, Robinson MR. Physicians' collaboration with chaplains: difficulties and benefits. *J Clin Ethics.* 1997;8:94–103.
2. Post SG, Puchalski C, Larson DB. Physician and patient spirituality: professional boundaries, competency, and ethics. *Ann Intern Med.* 2000;132:578–583.
3. Lo B, Quill T, Tulsky J. Discussing palliative care with patients. ACP-ASIM end-of-life care consensus panel. American College of Physicians-American Society of Internal Medicine. *Ann Intern Med.* 1999;130:744–749.
4. Chochinov HM, Wilson K, Enns M, et al. Desire for death in the terminally ill. *Am J Psychiatry.* 1995;152:1185–1191.
5. Chochinov HM, Tataryn D, Dudgeon D, et al. Will to live in the terminally ill. *Lancet.* 1999;354:816–819.
6. Back AL, Wallace JI, Starks HE, et al. Physician-assisted suicide and euthanasia in Washington state: patient requests and physician responses. *JAMA.* 1996;275:919–925.
7. Emanuel EJ, Fairclough DL, Daniels ER, et al. Euthanasia and physician-assisted suicide: attitudes and experiences of oncology patients, oncologists, and the public. *Lancet.* 1996;347:1805–1810.

8. Ganzini L, Nelson HD, Schmidt TA, et al. Physicians' experiences with the Oregon Death with Dignity Act. *N Engl J Med.* 2000;342:557–563.

9. Meier DE, Emmons CA, Wallenstein S, et al. A national survey of physician-assisted suicide and euthanasia in the United States. *N Engl J Med.* 1998:338:1193–1201.

10. Sullivan AD, Hedberg K, Fleming DW. Legalized physician-assisted suicide in Oregon: the second year. *N Engl J Med.* 2000;342:598–604.

11. Van der Maas PJ, Van Delden JJM, Pijnenborg L, et al. Euthanasia and other medical decisions concerning the end of life. *Lancet.* 1991;338:669–674.

12. Wilson KG, Scott JF, Graham ID, et al. Attitudes of terminally ill patients toward euthanasia and physician-assisted suicide. *Arch Intern Med.* 2000;160:2454–2460.

13. Chochinov HM, Wilson KG, Enns M, et al. Depression, hopelessness, and suicidal ideation in the terminally ill. *Psychosomatics.* 1998;39:366–370.

14. Breitbart W, Rosenfeld B, Pessin H, et al. Depression, hopelessness, and desire for hastened death in terminally ill cancer patients. *JAMA.* 2000;284:2907–2911.

15. Breitbart W, Rosenfeld B, Passik S. Interest in physician assisted suicide among ambulatory HIV infected patients. *Am J Psychiatry.* 1996;153:238–242.

16. Chochinov HM, Wilson KG, Enns M, et al. Prevalence of depression in the terminally ill: effects of diagnostic criteria and symptom threshold judgements. *Am J Psychiatry.* 1994;151:537–540.

17. Chochinov HM, Hack T, Hassard T, et al. Dignity in the terminally ill: a cross sectional cohort study. *Lancet.* 2002;360:2026–2030.

18. Chochinov HM, Hack T, McClement S, et al. Dignity in the terminally ill: an empirical model. *Soc Sci Med.* 2002;54:433–443.

19. Chochinov HM. Dignity conserving care: a new model for palliative care. *JAMA.* 2002;287:2253–2260.

6

Dignity. Dignity? Dignity!

As medicine evolves, so too does our thinking about clinical practice and the nature of our responsibility toward patients. Palliative care is no exception. When Dame Cicely Saunders founded the modern hospice movement nearly 60 years ago, her vision included attentiveness to physical, psychological, spiritual, and existential matters facing patients nearing death. This person-centered approach is succinctly captured in her famous adage, "You matter because you are you, and you matter to the end of your life. We will do all we can not only to help you die peacefully, but also to live until you die."

In the decades that followed, much attention was directed toward developing the science and clinical standards of practice, primarily focused on symptom management—pain, nausea, breathlessness, fatigue, depression, and anxiety, among others. Palliative care clinicians and clinician-scientists amassed evidence and experience, all forerunners of additional major achievements in the field, including the publication of the Oxford Textbook of Palliative Medicine *(now in its sixth edition),* The Handbook of Psychiatry in Palliative Medicine *(now in its third edition), and specialty journals such as the* Journal of Palliative Medicine, Journal of Pain and Symptom Management, *and* Palliative and Supportive Care. *In 1990 the World Health Organization recognized palliative care as a distinct specialty dedicated to relieving suffering and improving quality of life for patients with life-limiting illnesses or serious injuries. This led to establishing palliative care subspecialty training programs in various jurisdictions worldwide, under the banner of The Royal College of Physicians and Surgeons of Canada, The American Board of Medical Specialties, and the Accreditation Council for Graduate Medical Education, among many others.*

The evidentiary basis of contemporary palliative medicine is impressive. Clinicians have access to new and effective ways of ameliorating symptoms for patients who are suffering. I'll never forget watching Dr. Mike Harlos— a extraordinarily clinician and beloved colleague—attend to a woman during a pain crisis. He stepped away from ward rounds and, with various

In Search of Dignity. Harvey Max Chochinov, Oxford University Press. © Oxford University Press 2025.
DOI: 10.1093/9780197805145.003.0006

syringes and medications in hand, didn't leave her bedside (within the half hour as I recall) until she was resting comfortably. Truly awe-inspiring.

The article I am responding to by Dr. Andy Billings suggests there is a tension between the hard-fought identify of palliative medicine—and its evidence-based achievements—and my assertion that dignity-conserving care needs to be on our clinical radar and considered an overarching goal. Sadly, Andy died before I was able to discuss this with him. He was a good man, truly a pioneer who contributed so much to the discipline of palliative medicine. I think Andy would be pleased to see how the field has evolved in ways that are entirely consistent with Dame Cicely's original vision. Quality comprehensive palliative care requires attentiveness to the physical, psychological, spiritual, and existential dimensions of end-of-life experience. The science and the art of palliative are complementary, as are "care" and "caring." One without the other falls short on what palliative care can and should offer patients with health-related suffering.

Dignity. Dignity? Dignity! Harvey Max Chochinov. *Journal of Palliative Medicine*, 2008;11(5):674–675. Reprinted with permission from Mary Ann Liebert, Inc. publishers.

Dear Editor:

One might think, given how often I speak and write about dignity, that I suffer some strange variety of perseverative disorder. Such, however, is not the case.

Why then, do I—or more accurately, does our research team—go on about it? The primary incentive is that it just might be making a difference to how we understand and approach care for the dying. It is hard to imagine a more powerful motivation for sustaining, over nearly 20 years, our program of palliative care research.

In his editorial, Dr. Billings cautions the palliative care community not to rally itself "under the banner of dignity conservation"; that "dignity-preservation threatens to displace other goals of palliative medicine" and could possibly "elbow out our broader views of the goals of palliative care."[1] Let me try to reassure you, there is nothing to worry about.

Our segue into "dignity research" began with some published reports, documenting an association between considerations of hastened death and a loss of dignity.[2] Thus began our attempts to explicate this poorly understood, but seemingly life sustaining, idea. Dr. Billings asks if dignity is really important to patients, citing two studies where dignity did not rank highly on a list of dying patients expressed concerns. We too have reported that only a minority of the dying experience a marked or significant loss of sense of dignity.[1] However, among patients who no longer want to go on living, the association with dignity has been well articulated.[2,4] It would seem the importance of dignity becomes most transparent when it is threatened or undermined, just as the importance of pain becomes all-consuming when it is out of control.

Dr. Billings is also concerned that dignity lacks definitional specificity. His point is well taken, which is why, nearly 10 years ago, we published an empirically based model of dignity in the terminally ill.[5,6] We asked dying patients to articulate their notions of dignity, only to discover that it meant different things to different people. However, far from rendering the term dispensable, this data yielded an empirical model, delineating the multiplicity of issues and concerns falling under the rubric of dignity. It is this very breadth that provides the concept of dignity its potency to inform and improve palliative end-of-life care.

So what are some of the things that Dr. Billings thinks dignity will threaten or somehow displace? (I find it hard to imagine dignity in terms of sharp elbows, rather than seeing it, metaphorically, as a gentle touch.) He mentions "providing physical, emotional, social and spiritual support." Each of these are subsumed and carefully described within the dignity model; physical concerns falling under the theme, Illness Related Factors; emotional and spiritual support under the Dignity-Conserving Repertoire; and social issues under the theme coined the Social Dignity Inventory.[5] He also states that concepts like hope, growth, and dignity may not, in and of themselves, "yield a balanced view of patient and family values." As it happens, we have shown that Dignity Therapy, a brief individual psychological intervention based on the dignity model, provides an opportunity to reduce hopelessness and enhance a sense of meaning, purpose and dignity for patients nearing death.[7,8]

Dr. Billings subtly implies that it is rather simplistic to think we can ""conserve" [dignity] in a straight forward A-B-C-D fashion." The latter refers to a recent publication, in which I use our dignity research to introduce a framework, a mnemonic, describing the core values of medical professionalism, including kindness, humanity and respect.[9] Within this Dignity-Conserving

Care framework, "A" stands for attitude, that is, how the attitude of the health care provider can shape the patient's sense of dignity, perceived worth or self-value. Without data, which we provide in abundance, these words are perhaps little more than poetic, resonating with some, falling on deaf ears for others. The message about attitude is powerful. It says to anyone with patient contact, that they are a mirror into which patients look for some affirming reflection. "B" stands for behavior and how our behavior—providing someone undivided attention, not appearing rushed, a simple hand on the shoulder—can affirm patient dignity. The "C" of dignity-conserving care stands for compassion and describes how health care providers arrive at compassion; each at their own pace and in their own way, based on their own source of inspiration. Finally, "D" is for dialogue and the importance of conversations that affirm a patient's sense of personhood.

Is the A-B-C-D framework, as Dr. Billings implies, too simplistic? It is certainly true that probing the depths of human psychology and the nature of existential and spiritual suffering at end of life is extraordinarily complex and profoundly humbling. But how long must those of us working in the field complain about health care providers who "just don't seem to get it"? How many conversations will recount examples of insensitivity, poor judgment based on lack of empathy, clinical missteps that could have been avoided, if only a moment had been taken to see the person and not just the patient? Perhaps the ability to easily deliver our message has been hampered by an overemphasis on complexity. Why not, at the very least, try to offer a very simple, exceedingly intuitive, empirically based and highly memorable message. The A-B-C-Ds of dignity conserving care; your attitude, your behavior, your ability to feel compassion and engage in dialogue that acknowledges personhood are critical within the culture of health care. None of us is absolved from knowing the ABC's of critical care—airway, breathing, circulation. Why shouldn't there be a similar, basic mnemonic, defining core essential qualities of medical professionalism? Why not teach it to our students? Why not tell our non-palliative care colleagues that there is an important simple message, which might help them define core competencies, set standards, inform accreditation and reform curricula?

Are you still worried that an allegedly pugilistic dignity will knock out other core values and principles of palliative care? If all were allowed entry into the clinical arena, it is hard to imagine a single punch being thrown; what would be the point? And patients, their families and the profession of palliative care would of course emerge the winners. A metaphorically fanciful idea perhaps. The truth is, what I think about these issues matters little. What matters is listening to patients, doing careful research, and going where the data lead. And at least for now, it keeps leading me back to Dignity. Dignity? Dignity!

References

1. Billings A. Dignity. *J Palliat Med.* 2008;11:138–139.
2. Van Der Maas PJ, Van Delden JJ, Pijnenborg L, Looman CW. Euthanasia and other medical decisions concerning the end of life. *Lancet.* 1991;338:669–674.
3. Chochinov HM, Hack T, Hassard T, et al. Dignity in the terminally ill: a cross sectional, cohort study. *Lancet.* 2002;360:2026–2030.
4. Meier DE, Emmons CA, Wallenstein S, et al. A national survey of physician-assisted suicide and euthanasia in the United States. *N Engl J Med.* 1998;338:1193–1201.
5. Chochinov HM, Hack T, McClement S, et al. Dignity in the terminally ill: an empirical model. *Soc Sci Med.* 2002;54:433–443.
6. Chochinov HM. Dignity-conserving care—a new model for palliative care: helping the patient feel valued. *JAMA.* 2002;287:2253–2260.
7. Chochinov HM, Hack T, Hassard T, et al. Dignity therapy: a novel psychotherapeutic intervention for patients near the end of life. *J Clin Oncol.* 2005;23:5520–5525.
8. Chochinov HM. Dying, dignity, and new horizons in palliative end-of-life care. *CA Cancer J Clin.* 2006;56:84–103.
9. Chochinov HM. Dignity and the essence of medicine: the A, B, C & D of dignity-conserving care. *BMJ.* 2007;335:184–187.

7

Dignity, Memory, and Final Wishes of Dying Children

The first paper on Dignity Therapy appeared in the Journal of Clinical Oncology *nearly 20 years ago (Dignity Therapy: A novel psychotherapeutic intervention for patients nearing death.* J Clin Oncol. *2005;23:5520–5525). Since than there have been scores of publications and about a dozen systematic reviewers, affirming the utility of Dignity Therapy and its ever-expanding applications. Dignity Therapy was originally conceived as a palliative care intervention for adults nearing death. The Model of Dignity in the Terminally Ill, which is the theoretical basis of Dignity Therapy, emerged from studying older patients receiving palliative care, who, for the most part, were dying of advanced malignancies.*

Over time Dignity Therapy has been extended to other populations. There have been studies examining it in earlier-stage cancers, nonmalignant life-limiting conditions, neurodegenerative disorders, and other circumstances where death isn't imminent, such as patients with early-stage dementia or the frail elderly. Some researchers have examined the use of Dignity Therapy for patients with serious mental illness, and others for people dying in prisons. If there is a common denominator, it is using this legacy-based approach as a response to assaults on intactness of personhood. This certainly affirms that dying does not have a monopoly on the capacity to undermine sense of self.

This editorial about the utility of Dignity Therapy for children is one I wrote with my dear friend and colleague Dr. Miguel Julião. Aside from the creativity and sensitivity that has gone into considering Dignity Therapy for children, I am struck by how ideas placed in the public domain evolve over time and how talented people around the world use those ideas to shape and inform research and novel approaches to patient care. This is such an important part of the scientific process and reflects how meaningful

In Search of Dignity. Harvey Max Chochinov, Oxford University Press. © Oxford University Press 2025.
DOI: 10.1093/9780197805145.003.0007

innovation evolves in the service of meeting the needs of patients, young, less young, and old alike.

Dignity, Memory, and Final Wishes of Dying Children. Harvey Max Chochinov and Miguel Julião. *Journal of Palliative Medicine,* 2021;24(2):171–171. Reprinted with permission from Mary Ann Liebert, Inc. publishers.

Dear Editor:

Dignity therapy (DT) is one of the most studied brief psychotherapeutic interventions in palliative care today.[1] It enables patients nearing death to share memories, wisdom, hopes, wishes, and dreams with those who will soon grieve their loss. The key elements of DT are based on the Model of Dignity in the Terminally Ill[2]; and focus on important roles, accomplishments, and especially, the notion of generativity, which, according to developmental psychologist Erik Erikson, comprises leaving a lasting mark on the world and contributing to the next generation. Since the model is based on a cohort of older patients, largely with end-stage cancer, DT has exclusively been considered for dying adults. Given its ability to enhance end-of-life experience, the question is often raised as to its role among dying children.

Up until now, the answer has been, we simply have no evidence to suggest that DT might be an appropriate option for terminally ill children. Julião et al. reported a revised version of DT for adolescence, positing several metaphors and tasks to make it more developmentally appropriate.[3] Although this adaptation was based on input from a qualified expert panel, it has yet to be implemented. Schuelke and Rubenstein's study offers important insights, suggesting that DT, revised to meet the needs of dying children and adolescents, has a place within the pediatric palliative care therapeutic armamentarium.[4] Although all participants reported positive outcomes, the revisions needed to make DT suitable in this context are worthy of reflection.

Shortly after the death of nine-year-old Madeline "Maddie" Dibello, members of her immediate family took part in DT by way of proxy. Afterward they reported feeling peaceful, with the mother indicating that the final document reflected how the family felt about her child. Other studies have described DT by proxy, with health care providers and family members of patients with dementia reporting heightened sense of dignity, meaning, and appreciation of who the resident was as a person.[5]

Upon completing his DT, 19-year-old Alex Unger had his sister create the cover art for his generativity document. This is consistent with Julião et al. who suggested that art, photography, video, or audio recordings can embellish legacy documents of adolescent patients.[3] Sixteen-year-old Miracle Akbar held a party at which she read her generativity document, whereas Shahd Shahroor had her document translated into her family's native tongue of Arabic and took great pride in the document being used for educational purposes. Although perhaps motivated by altruism, her reaction also suggests comfort in knowing her story will be told.

By adding art, video, photography, and similar creative embellishments, young people—or their proxies—are able to engage in a process that provides lasting testimony to their lives. Perhaps the one thing that all these cases illustrate is that being remembered, and the ability to appreciate the notion of being held in the memory of those left behind, is critical when considering DT for child and adolescent patients. By enabling the preservation of memory, DT can help fulfill the final wishes of children nearing death.

References

1. Chochinov HM. *Dignity Therapy: Final Words for Final Days*. Oxford University Press; 2012.
2. Chochinov HM, Hack T, McClement S, et al. Dignity in the terminally ill: a developing empirical model. *Soc Sci Med*. 2002;54:433–443.
3. Julião M, Antunes B, Santos A, et al. Adapting the Portuguese dignity question framework for adolescents: ages 10–18. *Palliat Support Care*. 2020;18:199–205.
4. Schuelke T, Rubenstein J. Dignity therapy in pediatrics: a case series. *Palliat Med Rep*. 2020;1(1):156–160.
5. Chochinov HM, Cann B, Cullihall K, et al. Dignity therapy: a feasibility study of elders in long-term care. *J Palliat Support Care*. 2012;10:3–15.

8

Death, Dying, and Dignity in the Time of the COVID-19 Pandemic

There is a photograph etched in my mind of my wife, Michelle, at the height of the pandemic. She is standing outside of the first-floor room window of the personal care home where her 95-year-old cousin Joyce spent her final months of life in isolation. In the photograph, Michelle is holding a cellphone trying to speak with Joyce. Joyce's image can faintly be seen beyond the windowpane. Looking carefully, it appears she is sitting in her chair next to the window, and someone—a nurse or perhaps a healthcare aide—is helping her pick up the call.

For me, this image symbolizes so much of what the COVID-19 pandemic was about: what it did to people, especially people who were older and more vulnerable, and what it took away from us all. It is difficult to see Joyce in this photograph, and of course, impossible to touch her. That experience, worldwide, was COVID's doing. It made it difficult to connect with people in ways we previously took for granted. It took away our ability to be present and to express love, affection, and support in ways that felt natural and intuitive, leaving fear and lingering regret in its wake. Joyce died alone (mercifully, we were called in the day before to say our goodbyes). Her funeral, with a mere handful of attendees, including pallbearers, was a shadow of what she deserved.

In this article, Death, Dying, and Dignity in the Time of the COVID-19 Pandemic, *I share some early reflections on the havoc wrought by COVID-19 and the dire assault on human dignity. The pandemic traumatized the world in ways that are difficult to articulate, with reverberations still being felt to this very day. In the fall of 2022, our research team launched a series of studies examining how dying patients, their families, and healthcare providers were being affected by COVID-19. Our first study, which was focused on the experience of patients nearing death, reported, "While infection control insists on measures based on separation and isolation, the basic human need for love, dignity, and care approaching death insists on*

In Search of Dignity. Harvey Max Chochinov, Oxford University Press. © Oxford University Press 2025.
DOI: 10.1093/9780197805145.003.0008

proximity and connection.[a] *Our next publication examined how health-care providers attending to dying patients were affected by the pandemic and the ways in which it undermined their ability to provide dignity-conserving palliative care.*[b] *We also recently reported on virtual funerals and the extent to which they were able to fulfill the needs of bereft families during the pandemic.*[c]

We are now completing several other papers based on this program of research, including one examining personhood in the intensive care unit setting, where families were not allowed to be with their dying relatives due to public health restrictions. We conducted this program of research knowing this isn't the first, nor will it be the last, time the world will face cataclysmic health crises. Studies exploring the effects of COVID-19 on death, dying, and dignity will help the world be better prepared.

Death, Dying, and Dignity in the Time of the COVID-19 Pandemic. Harvey Max Chochinov, James Bolton, and Jitender Sareen. *Journal of Palliative Medicine*, 2020;23(10):1294–1295. Reprinted with permission from Mary Ann Liebert, Inc. publishers.

If the first casualty of war is truth, the first casualty of coronavirus disease (COVID-19) for patients nearing death is human dignity. Although the pandemic has claimed ~6800 Canadian lives, ~60,000 people have died in Canada since the World Health Organization declared the novel coronavirus (COVID-19) outbreak a global pandemic.[d] Given the insidious nature of this virus, care for patients dying of any cause has been distorted in ways previously thought unimaginable. Because of public health restrictions, patients are dying alone. Even for the sickest of sick, whether they are dying in palliative care units, medical or surgical wards, intensive care units, hospices, or long-term care facilities, limited visitation polices are being strictly enforced.

---

[a] Pirzada S, Papineau K, Pankratz L, et al. The first casualty of COVID-19 for patients nearing death was human dignity: understanding the experience of palliative care patients during the COVID-19 pandemic. *Death Stud.* 2024;49(6):699–713.

[b] Pankratz L, Gill G, Pirzada S, et al. "It took so much of the humanness away": health care professional experiences providing care to dying patients during COVID-19. *Death Stud.* 2024;48:706–718.

[c] Wilson L, Gill G, Pirzada S, et al. Together, alone: personal experiences of virtual funeral attendance during the COVID-19 global pandemic. *Death Stud.* 2024 Oct 7:1–13.

[d] As of April 2024, close to 60,000 Canadians had died as a result of COVID-19.

The primary contact these dying patients have is with health care providers, with whom touch can only be experienced through layers of latex, eye contact through layers of goggles and plastic shields, and human presence through layers of anxiety, caution, and fear.

A recent systematic review reported that hospitalized patients placed in isolation for medical reasons are more likely to experience depression, anxiety, anger, and loss of self-esteem; health care providers spend less time with them, impacting patient safety with an eightfold difference in adverse events related to supportive care failures.[1] Other studies have shown that loneliness is a risk factor for mental disorders, such as depression, anxiety, adjustment disorder, chronic distress, and insomnia. Our own research has shown that lack of social support, symptom distress, and not feeling valued or respected can undermine a dying patient's sense of dignity.[2] Those who are isolated or avoided are especially vulnerable, inclined to feel that they may not only *have* a contagion, but that they *are* a contagion.

Families barred visitation are denied the opportunity to bear witness, advocate for optimal health care, and must forgo final goodbyes. Not having access to their dying loved ones may put families at risk for complicated grief. Not being able to follow a path of least regret leaves many questions unanswered. Did their loved ones receive the best care possible? Were they in pain? What were they thinking about in those final weeks and days of life? Was someone with them when they died? As if that were not enough, the pandemic has meant that families must forgo community rituals of mourning. Funerals have been reduced to graveside services of 5 to 10 people, with live streaming alternatives the only option for those wishing to virtually pay their respects. After an outbreak of severe acute respiratory syndrome-related coronavirus in 2002–2004, the SARS commission final report noted that "those left behind had no opportunity to confront the reality of death and to honor the life of the deceased" (p. 943), with the proviso that "funeral rites must obviously carry lower priority than the need to contain the virulent public health threat" (p. 942).[3] These distortions in the process of death and dying foreshadow similar distortions in the process of grieving and could mean higher risk of various psychiatric morbidities such as depression, anxiety, post-traumatic stress disorder, and suicidal ideation.

The pandemic has seen health care providers being forced to engage in what some have called *impoverished care*, wherein the obligations toward patient care must be weighed against obligations for self-protection and that of one's family. A recent study out of China described the experiences of physicians and nurses with no infectious disease expertise recruited to care for patients with COVID-19.[4] They reported exhaustion due to heavy workloads and protective gear, fear of becoming infected and infecting others, feeling powerless to handle patients' conditions, accompanied by a sense of being fully responsible for patients' well-being. The pandemic has seen health care providers confronting multiple concurrent deaths, moral distress, helplessness, and burnout. It is too early to say what complications, such as depression, Posttraumatic Distress Disorder (PTSD), substance abuse, or suicide, will manifest.

With dignity under assault, now is the time to be mindful of the ABCD's of dignity-conserving care: A for attitude, B for behavior, C for compassion, and D for dialogue.[2] Our research has shown that the way dying patients perceive themselves to be seem, reflective of health care provider *attitude* toward them, is the most ardent predictor of maintaining dignity. Clinicians must be mindful that their outlook on patients shapes every clinical encounter. Changing attitudes means changing perceptions. Something as simple as the patient's photograph on their bedside table can remind us of who they are as a person, over and above whatever medical ailment brought them to our attention. The *behavior* component of dignity-conserving care must always be predicated on kindness and respect. Although behavior includes all acts and how one conducts oneself toward the patient, it begins with something as simple as "taking a seat." A randomized control trial reported that sitting instead of standing at the bedside can have significant impact on patient satisfaction, compliance, and provider–patient rapport, and that patients perceive their provider as being present at their bedside longer when sitting.[5]

Compassion (the C of dignity-conserving care) has been described as *a virtuous response that seeks to address the suffering and needs of a person through relational understanding and action*.[6] Compassion demands action to mitigate patient suffering. Whether it is bringing a glass of water, helping them change a television channel, finessing their medication, or listening to them (the perfect action for someone yearning to be heard), compassion can obviate our sense of helplessness or therapeutic nihilism. Dialogue (the D of dignity-conserving care) refers to the conversations and communication we have with patients in the service of affirming personhood.

Our research group has developed and tested a simple question coined *The Patient Dignity Question (PDQ)*, which asks patients, "What do I need to know about you as a person to take the best care of you possible?"[7] In a cohort of 126 palliative care participants, 97% gave permission to have a brief summary of their PDQ response placed on their chart, 99% said they would recommend it to other patients in their circumstances, and 85% felt the information was important for their health care provider to know. Of the 137 health care providers who gave feedback, most indicated that they learned something new from the PDQ, that it affected them emotionally, and heightened their sense of empathy and connectedness with their patients. We also found an association between receptiveness to information gleaned from the PDQ and health care provider job satisfaction, meaning in life, and overall personal empathy. Another tool we have developed, TIME (This Is Me), provides clinicians a somewhat more structured and detailed alternative to the PDQ as a means of eliciting personhood. In a study of personal care home residents, TIME was reported to heighten sense of dignity, change how others might see or appreciate them, and convey what matters to them, including their worries and concerns.[8]

Dying with dignity has been a problem during the COVID-19 pandemic, a problem that transcends national and international borders and one where there is no safe haven or end in sight. Research is needed into dignity-conserving care, ensuring that, wherever patients are dying, dignity does not fall prey to this insidious virus.

References

1. Abad C, Fearday A, Safdar N. Adverse effects of isolation in hospitalized patients: a systematic review. *J Hosp Infect.* 2010;76:97–102.
2. Chochinov HM. Dignity and the essence of medicine: the A, B, C and D of dignity conserving care. *Br Med J.* 2007;335:184–187.
3. Funerals and the suffering of families. In: *SARS Commission Final Report; Vol. III: Spring of Fear.* archives.gov.on.ca/en/e_records/sars/report/v3-pdf/Vol3Chp5v.pdf
4. Liu Q, Luo D, Guo Q, et al. The experiences of health-care providers during the COVID-19 crisis in China: a qualitative study. *Lancet Glob Health.* 2020;8:e790–e798.
5. Swayden KJ, Anderson KK, Connelly LM, et al. Effect of sitting vs. standing on perception of provider time at bed-side: a pilot study. *Patient Educ Couns.* 2012;86:166–171.
6. Sinclair S, Norris JM, McConnell SJ, et al. Compassion: a scoping review of the healthcare literature. *BMC Palliat Care.* 2016;15:6.
7. Chochinov HM, McClement S, Hack T, et al. Eliciting personhood within clinical practice: effects on patients, families and health care providers. *J Pain Symptom Manage.* 2015;49:974–980.
8. Pan L, Chochinov HM, Thompson G, et al. The TIME questionnaire: a tool for eliciting personhood and enhancing dignity in nursing homes. *Geriatr Nurs.* 2016;37:273–277.

SECTION 3
PERSONHOOD AND ATTENDING TO SUFFERING

9

Why is Being a Patient a Difficult Pill to Swallow?

Most of my writing has been for professional audiences, but at some point it dawned on me that these messages about the "human side of medicine" might resonate with the public. After all, the experience of illness is universal: all of us have been, currently are, or will inevitably become patients or those caring for them. Illnesses may be short-lived, only requiring acute medical care, or may become more frequent and chronic, which means we will take up longer-term residence in this vulnerable space.

The physical challenges of patienthood vary based on the illness and its expressions that bring someone to medical attention. My research has focused on the psychological and existential challenges of patienthood, including how it can undermine feeling like "I'm still me." I recently saw a gentleman who was considering medical assistance in dying. His illness had taken away much of his capacity to do things that were fundamental to his sense of self and personal identity. When I asked him why he thought he needed to die, his response was, "I'm not me anymore."

When illness or medical concerns are minor or time-limited, assaults on personhood are more easily withstood. If you're kept waiting for a medical appointment, if your doctor uses a brusque tone, or if you have to submit to a physical examination, most people can tap into their coping reserves without feeling substantively diminished. But when sickness becomes significant or protracted, our resilience diminishes and our sensitivity to these assaults increases.

I've spent much of my career sensitizing healthcare professionals to these critical dynamics and the power they wield, shaping each clinical encounter. Patients also need to understand the complexities of being healthcare recipients so they can assert their needs, express their individuality, and not get lost in a medical system that can sometimes feel dehumanizing. This was my motivation for writing this piece.

In Search of Dignity. Harvey Max Chochinov, Oxford University Press. © Oxford University Press 2025. DOI: 10.1093/9780197805145.003.0009

Why is Being a Patient a Difficult Pill to Swallow? by Harvey Max Chochinov. An earlier version of this essay first appeared in *Toronto Star* on January 27th, 2023.

While being treated for an aggressive hematologic cancer, the former Head of a Department of Medicine at a large teaching hospital told me he wished he could hang a sign on his headboard, reading P-I-P: Previously-Important-Person. Despite extraordinary achievements, skills, credentials, and status, being a patient made him feel like an amalgam of parts; limbs, bodily fluids, organs, and orifices, all now suspect, some more wayward than others—and most, for his taste, far too readily on display.

Why is being a patient such a difficult pill to swallow?

Besides whatever concern or ailment brings you to seek medical care, there is something about the very nature of being a patient that deeply rankles. Whether trying to arrange a medical appointment, waiting to be seen in a clinic or hospital, or being examined under the watchful gaze of a healthcare provider, being a patient disrupts our sense of intactness, gnawing away like an existential termite.

At its core is the erosion of personhood and a feeling that identity is under attack, threatening to displace the essence of who we really are.

It doesn't have to be this way. Our sense of who we are as people is highly individualized, based on personal experiences and relationships; affiliations, attitudes, culture, beliefs, abilities; opportunities and connections; inclinations and foibles. In other words, who you are as a person is highly specific and unique; never has there been, nor ever again, will there be one exactly like you. Being a patient, on the other hand, is based entirely on things that are generic.

Bodily parts are supposed to behave in exact and predictable ways, irrespective of who their owner happens to be. With all due respect, whether prince(cess) or pauper, poet or pilot, your bits and bobs are pretty much identical, in form and function, relative to everyone else's.

And herein lies the problem with being a patient. The moment we enter the healthcare system, the focus of attention shifts from who we are, to the ailment or problem we are now facing. This shift puts identity in jeopardy.

A long-time dialysis nurse once told me she eventually came to think of patients as kidneys on legs. Patienthood eclipses personhood, casting a shadow that undermines the essence of who we are. This is bad for patients and their families; it is also bad for healthcare providers since emotional disconnection and objectification of patients is a harbinger for professional burnout.

One approach designed to decrease this kind of existential trauma is beginning to take hold, coined the Patient Dignity Question (PDQ). The PDQ asks patients, "What do I need to know about you as a person to take the best care of you possible?" This question forms the basis of a brief five-to-ten-minute conversation, focused on personhood. What matters to you? What are your core beliefs? What or who are you most worried about? What roles and relationships matter most?

In answering the PDQ, patients are being asked how they want to be seen or understood as a person by their healthcare team. These conversations are summarized into a few paragraphs, and with the patient's approval, placed on their medical chart.

While mostly used in patients with serious illness, the PDQ is relevant across all of medicine.

Whether you are being seen for routine medical care, or find yourself moving towards the end of life, or somewhere in between, who you are and acknowledgement of who you are as a person, matters. And the things that people disclose by way of the PDQ profoundly change the way healthcare providers see them. I'm a survivor of childhood abuse. My son is battling cancer. I am afraid to die alone. I am a former department head of medicine.

During the COVID-19 pandemic, the daughter of a woman on a ventilator in intensive care shared that her mother had survived the likely murder of her first child and was a spiritual leader in her community. She said that responding to the PDQ gave her a way of letting the healthcare team know that her mother "was no ordinary person."

These kind of disclosures profoundly and forever change the healthcare provider's lens, bringing an appreciation of who patients are as persons, above and beyond whatever ailment brought them to medical attention. This is good for healthcare providers, helping stave off emotional indifference that can lead to professional burnout, while restoring human connection with the potential for them to be more whole themselves.

It is also good for patients and families, ensuring that patienthood doesn't overshadow personhood.

Being a patient is hard, especially when it undermines your feeling that you are still you. That, it turns out, is the hardest pill to swallow of all.

10

Michael J. Fox Gives Patients Hope There May Be a Place Illness Doesn't Touch

I have long been intrigued by the idea of places illness cannot touch. Much of my clinical work over the past few decades has been with patients facing imminent death. While various losses and disabilities are an expected part of that journey, I am struck by how patients retain core aspects of themselves. Despite advanced illness, patients are usually able to tell me what matters to them, who and what they care about, how they experience the world and their place in it, and the details of their lives and connections with people, especially those who mean the most to them.

This idea of "places illness cannot touch" has important implications for how patients navigate illness when it assaults their individual autonomy and sense of self. Illness often disrupts our ability "to do," as distinct from our ability "to be." "Being" equates to essence, which captures the idea of who we are and what we are, as distinct from what we do or what we have or can achieve. And being matters. The Book of Common Prayer *reads, "If I am to stand up, help me to stand bravely. If I am to sit still, help me to sit quietly. If I am to lie low, help me to do it patiently. And if I am to do nothing, let me do it gallantly." The very idea that doing nothing can be gallant means being has value. Even in the absence of doing, people's lives matter. Providing them with affirmation—which is something my research has explored in various forms and settings—allows patients to experience themselves as being valued and to see themselves as having enduring worth.*

Which is why I found the Netflix documentary about Michael J. Fox deeply moving. It is essentially a story about a man who, despite facing illness and loss, is able to maintain his sense of self. It's little wonder that it was released under the title Still.

In Search of Dignity. Harvey Max Chochinov, Oxford University Press. © Oxford University Press 2025.
DOI: 10.1093/9780197805145.003.0010

Michael J. Fox Gives Patients Hope There May Be a Place Illness Doesn't Touch by Harvey Max Chochinov. An earlier version of this essay first appeared in *Globe and Mail* on July 7, 2023.

Still: A Michael J. Fox Movie was recently released by Apple TV+ and provides a ringside seat to the daily, formidable challenges facing the actor since he was diagnosed with Parkinson's disease more than 30 years ago.

There is, of course, tremendous irony in this movie's title, given Parkinson's disease, a non-curable neurodegenerative disease that affects well over six million people around the world, denies those afflicted the ability to keep still. As was the case with Mr. Fox, it often begins with a tremor in one hand, which over time progresses to generalized slowness of movement, resting tremors and difficulties with balance resulting in falls. Stillness becomes a distant memory; a resting state of immobility that is no longer part of one's repertoire. The film's title has other resonances, including the idea of calmness and feelings of inner peace.

The closest we see Mr. Fox demonstrate that kind of stillness comes when he speaks about or is seen with his family. In those instances, he doesn't seem to be contemplating the next quick-witted one-liner or embodying the part of iconic actor or international Parkinson's spokesperson and philanthropist.

In one particularly poignant scene, while expressing frustration with his physiotherapy routine, his personal trainer reminds him that he doesn't always have to be Michael J. Fox. In other words, he's told it is okay to let go of the public image, and the responsibilities and expectations that go along with it. It is one of the few times his sadness emerges without him attempting to deflect away from the pain. Rather than a clever rejoinder, he chooses silence.

There are times when finding inner peace within the midst of deteriorating health requires confronting anguish. Like grief, responding to illness-related losses can't be outrun or circumvented. But that kind of being in the moment engagement, painful though it may be, can bring about a kind of calm that people sometimes speak of in terms of healing.

Mr. Fox says, "I couldn't be present in my life until I found this thing happened to me that made me present in every moment of my life because it was shaking me awake." Parkinson's disease, without any benevolent intent whatsoever, forced Michael J. Fox to make room for Michael.

I've spent the entirety of my career as a psychiatrist working with patients facing life-threatening and life-limiting conditions. My research shows that "no longer feeling like the person you once were" can crush a person's sense of dignity and sap the desire for life itself. The challenge for patients facing illness-related losses is trying to locate and preserve core elements of self that define who they are.

Mr. Fox says, despite his illness, "I love my mind and I love the places it takes me." I suspect those places haven't changed much over the course of his lifetime; they are places teeming with wit, imagination, and fun; and they are places where Parkinson's doesn't occupy any significant real estate. When asked to imagine his life a decade or two from now, Mr. Fox responds, with perfect, impeccable timing, "I'll either be cured, or I'll be a pickle!" That sounds *exactly* like Michael J. Fox.

I remember looking after an older woman with metastatic breast cancer many years ago. She was the matriarch of her family, and as I recall, ruled with an iron fist. Even as she lay on her deathbed, with a single wag of her finger, her family would jump into action. While dying broke her body and diminished her capacity, in spirit, she remained entirely herself, intact, formidable to the very end.

Parkinson's disease hasn't been able to occupy those extraordinary places within Mr. Fox, allowing him to maintain a sense that he's still the same person.

For many people confronting enormous health challenges, remaining oneself is directly linked to meaning and purpose. As Mr. Fox puts it, "I wanted to be in the world and not take this and retreat from the world." In so doing, he has made the world a better place, through his philanthropy—raising more than $2 billion for Parkinson's research—through his mobilization of the Parkinson's community, and now, with *Still*, through his honesty and transparency.

By showing us, unflinchingly, what Parkinson's can and can't break, he has given patients hope that there may be a place within themselves where they might take refuge, a place that illness mightn't touch. This may allow them to get back to a future imbued with meaning, purpose and hope.

For that, we are all collectively in Mr. Fox's debt—still.

11

Depression Is a Liar

This piece could only have been written by someone who has experienced depression. The details of that painful time are well known to those closest to me, and, for everyone else, the details don't matter. I just hope the insights gleaned from that psychological nightmare—long since in my rearview mirror—are of value to anyone who has been, is, or may become depressed.

Depression Is a Liar by Harvey Max Chochinov. An earlier version of this essay first appeared in *Globe and Mail* on May 3rd, 2023.

In February, just a few months after being elected to the United States Senate, Pennsylvania politician John Fetterman entered a treatment program for depression. In an interview with CBS News show *Sunday Morning* last month, he recounted suffering a stroke in May 2022, then fighting through a grueling Senate race that severely impacted his mental health. "You may have won," he recalled thinking, "but depression can absolutely convince you that you actually lost."

That's because depression is a liar.

Depression tells you you're not good enough. It whispers in your ear that you are flawed, that you are letting everyone down and that your life really doesn't matter. When things are particularly bad, depression seems to be shouting these lies from the rooftops.

Depression sets a passing grade on your life that is unattainable, and so, inevitably, depression tells you that you are failing. It leaves you feeling like the person you once were, or the person you think you need to be, is broken. This idea of "brokenness" or "fractured personhood" explains how depression tries to convince you to destroy yourself—why ending your life seems to be a way out. We try to eliminate the things we hate. Depression makes you believe your life is permanently shattered, and suicide offers a way of destroying the person you can no longer tolerate.

In Search of Dignity. Harvey Max Chochinov, Oxford University Press. © Oxford University Press 2025.
DOI: 10.1093/9780197805145.003.0011

Depression isn't concerned about logic, nor does it set rational expectations. I recall a physician who took his own life after his sibling died of the very disease in which he specialized. Depression, no doubt, convinced him he should have been able to save his sibling, and he, in turn, destroyed the person he somehow felt was responsible for not delivering a cure. The trauma of losing his sibling found him facing the limitations of what was possible, to which depression responded, "You should have been able to do more."

The nature of trauma—whether physical, emotional or spiritual—has the capacity to shatter your sense of being in control. Irrespective of the type of trauma you encounter, including being a witness to trauma, the result is a heightened risk of suicide.

But why is this the case?

Those experiencing physical or sexual assault discover that they can be overpowered, leaving them feeling fragile and weak. Those experiencing intimate partner violence or child abuse discover that familial connections don't necessarily protect them from violence, leaving them feeling defenseless. Those who are imprisoned learn that they cannot will themselves free, leaving them feeling trapped. The bereft discover that love can't protect those they cherish from the ravages of illness or calamity, leaving them feeling helpless. And those bearing witness to trauma learn that their abhorrence and horror carry no sway whatsoever, leaving them feeling like impotent bystanders.

Feeling fragile, weak, defenseless, trapped, helpless or impotent in the wake of trauma is at complete odds with the person they once were or the person they want to be. And so, in directing their rage inward, they destroy the person they deem broken, fractured and unworthy of living.

Depression will try to convince you that you are beyond help, and that no words or advice or insight will loosen its pathological grip. Escaping this psychological monster won't happen by trying to fulfill its insurmountable expectations; that will only cause additional torment, having you chase a finish line that is forever moving further down the track. This will make you feel inadequate, flawed—like you are failing; hence, playing right into depression's hand.

Like many who encounter depression, I suspect Mr. Fetterman will emerge from this experience feeling humbled—acutely aware of his own flaws and limitations.

But here is the truth. Listen carefully, even though depression will try to tell you otherwise. Those perceived flaws and limitations have nothing to do with failing, but rather are simply part of being human. All humans are vulnerable and mortal. All human beings stumble and struggle and eventually yield to forces beyond their control.

For everyone, and without exception, personhood can fracture and life, at times, leaves us feeling broken. Leonard Cohen wrote, "There is a crack in everything, that's how the light gets in." That light is our glorious, fragile, collective humanity.

Depression, being an incessant liar, wants to hide that truth, intent to keep you languishing in the dark.

May the light get in once again.

12

The Platinum Rule

A New Standard for Person-Centered Care

Doing research has always felt like following a thread. From the time this work began, I have been intrigued by and committed to chasing that thread wherever it might lead. Questions about why people with advanced illness might lose their desire to live led to new insights about depression and the nature of hope. This segued into studies focused on dignity and its powerful influence on sustaining people in the throes of advanced illness. Next came a deep dive into the psychological, existential, and spiritual complexities of patients approaching death, and the discovery that the tone of care and the healthcare provider's gaze can shape clinical encounters and patients' perceptions of dignity and sense of feeling affirmed.

We went on to explore how to influence the way healthcare providers see their patients, which meant developing approaches such as Dignity Therapy, the Patient Dignity Question, the ABCDs of Dignity-Conserving Care, and the Patient Dignity Inventory. All were designed to put per-sonhood on the clinical radar, offering clinicians a clearer picture of who patients are as whole persons. Although these approaches are meant to in-fluence what clinicians see, they do not change the intrinsic nature of the healthcare provider's lens.

Different clinicians can observe the same patient and yet see things quite differently. This suggests there is something about the nature of their indi-vidual gaze that shapes perceptions. Anaïs Nin wrote, "We see the world not as it is, but as we are." This manifests most dramatically when there are vast differences between the lived experiences of patients and those of their healthcare providers. In those instances, clinicians can't reliably use themselves to gauge what patients might want or need. Hence the Golden Rule—Do unto others as you would want done unto yourself—must yield to the Platinum Rule, which I explain in the next two articles.

Relatively early into the COVID-19 pandemic, I began exploring how social media can be applied in academia. I soon discovered that LinkedIn

In Search of Dignity. Harvey Max Chochinov, Oxford University Press. © Oxford University Press 2025.
DOI: 10.1093/9780197805145.003.0012

and Twitter are powerful communication tools, with a dazzling capacity for knowledge dissemination. Posting what I publish on those two platforms has become part of my routine. When the first article on the Platinum Rule came out in June 2022, I posted it with a note saying it provided some interesting insights on compassion, clinician bias, and person-centered care. Within 24 hours there were over 20,000 impressions. Within the month, I had been contacted by colleagues from opposite ends of the country, telling me they'd attended meetings or seminars about EDI (equity, diversity, and inclusiveness) in which the Platinum Rule had been cited. And then, to my utter amazement, in February 2023, Scientific American *published an editorial by Claudia Wallis titled "Better Patient Care Calls for a 'Platinum Rule' to Replace the Golden One"!*

It really is extraordinary where following a thread can take you, and how quickly what it reveals can spread.

The Platinum Rule: A New Standard for Person-Centered Care. Harvey Max Chochinov. *Journal of Palliative Medicine,* 2022;25(6):854–856. Reprinted with permission from Mary Ann Liebert, Inc. publishers.

Abstract

How decisions are made and patients cared for are often guided by the Golden Rule, which would have us treat patients as we would want to be treated in similar circumstances. But when patients' lived experiences and outlooks deviate substantively from our own, we stop being a reliable barometer of their needs, values, and goals. Inaccurate perceptions of their suffering and our personal biases may lead to distorted compassion, marked by an attitude of pity and therapeutic nihilism. In those instances, The Platinum Rule, which would have us consider *doing unto patients as they would want done unto themselves,* may be a more appropriate standard for achieving optimal person-centered care. This means knowing who patients are as persons, hence guiding treatment decisions and shaping a tone of care based on compassion and respect.

＊＊＊＊＊

Bert was a kind 74-year-old, happily married gentleman and father of five children. He had smoked cigarettes for a few decades, but had quit years ago, yet had presented with a cancer in his mouth. He underwent a large surgery that left him hoarse and disfigured. He was unable to swallow and depended on a gastrostomy tube for his feedings. Chemotherapy and radiation took their turns in causing more difficulties with nausea and some painful radiation effects.

Eventually the cancer recurred. More chemotherapy did not affect the tumour, and radiation was given with palliative intent. He began to have more pain, and at that point, one of his oncologists sat down with him and his wife and told them that he likely had little time to live, that his tumour was most likely going to progress quickly, and that his last days would become much more difficult, with increasing pain. The oncologist suggested that he might consider MAiD (Medical Assistance in Dying), to avoid what was sure to be a time of significant suffering.

Bert and his wife were a religious couple who had relied on prayer and the community around them to get them through over the years. They could not agree to MAiD. It was just not on their list of potential options. When he met with the palliative care consultant, he was having increasing pain, which was felt to have a large neuropathic component. A mix of gabapentin and small doses of methadone helped to reduce his pain to a very manageable level. The addition of immunotherapy by another oncologist resulted in a surprisingly good outcome, and now 6 months later, while still depending on gastrostomy feedings, he is frequently out in the garden, watering and weeding, and hoping to take part in harvest. He recently indicated his quality of life was excellent.[1]

The Golden Rule—*do unto others as you would have them do unto you*—conveys deep wisdom, which can be found in some form in many religious and ethical traditions. In medicine this means treating patients and families the way we would want to be treated or would want our loved ones to be treated in similar circumstances. The Golden Rule is based on the idea of reciprocity and being able to see ourselves in others. *If I were that patient, how would I want to be treated? What if this was my spouse, my child, my parent or sibling, how would I want them to be treated?* In most instances adherence to The Golden Rule leads to healthcare decisions and clinical attitudes that are compassionate and embrace the essence of person-centered care.

The Golden Rule however has its limitations, as it requires some overlap between how we see ourselves and how others see themselves. So long as the patient's values and priorities align with our own, we can infer their needs based on how we would want to be treated in their situation. The more our worldview and lived experience deviates from theirs, the more the Golden Rule begins to unravel. *How would I want to be treated if I were that old? If*

I were that dependent? Or that disabled, disfigured, marginalized, or disease ridden? Our own biases and perceptions of current, and the possibility of future, suffering can lead to attitudes that are tone deaf and decisions that are discordant with patients' perceptions, values, and goals.

What happens when, from an alleged vantagepoint of beneficence, we perceive someone to be suffering, based on how we imagine we would suffer in their situation? Unconscious bias can influence the way we process patient information, affecting our behaviour, interactions and decision-making.[2] A sense of therapeutic nihilism and clinical passivity can set in, a feeling that nothing is worth trying and certain lives may not be worth preserving, leading us to withhold treatment, perhaps forgo diagnostic tests and *let nature take its course.* Inferring we would not want to live this way, *distorted compassion*—that is, compassion based on tainted or inaccurate perceptions of another person's suffering—can lead to ostensibly well intended advice, actions or inactions that may be completely at odds with what the patient really wants. Rather than feeling that they have been heard, distorted compassion can result in patients feeling devalued, misunderstood, and further demoralized at the very hands of those who are meant to help.

Catherine Frazee, a preeminent disability rights advocate who lives with spinal muscular atrophy, says, "having to wear diapers and drooling are highly stigmatized departures from what is expected of adult bodies. Those of us who deviate from these norms experience social shame and stigma that erodes resilience and increases vulnerably. The more deeply these stigmatized accounts are embedded in our discourse and social policy, the more deeply virulent social prejudice takes hold within our culture.... What assurance can we offer that the physician who treat these adults at end-of-life will not stand at their bedside with horror or revulsion in his heart?"[3] Adhering to the Golden Rule, we may find ourselves responding with pity and implicit or explicit encouragement for patients to *let go*, despite their determination to *hang on*.

The *Platinum Rule,* which would have us consider *doing unto patients as they would want done unto themselves*, offers a standard that is more likely to result in treatment decisions that are consistent with patients' personal needs and objectives. *Doing unto* as per the Platinum Rule implicates not only clinical decisions, but treating patients—as in acting towards them—as they would want to be treated. This means establishing a care tenor that is informed by asking what we need to know about them as a person to take the best care of them possible.[4] This kind of sensitivity to personhood increases the likelihood that our responses are personalized and genuinely compassionate. And when stated preferences are less certain, it is important to explore their and their family's values to inform treatment recommendations. Deep inquiry is needed from a position of cultural humility, which emphasizes "that [healthcare providers] must acknowledge the experiential lens through which they view the world and that their view is not nearly as extensive, open, or dynamic as they might perceive."[2] This approach requires the development of self-awareness as a critical step in achieving mindfulness for others.[5] Of course, not all patient preferences can or should be accommodated, especially when they are driven by nihilistic self-loathing (*I don't want anything*), or motivated by expectations that exceed any objective reality (*I want everything*). Even then, it is important to understand their wishes, and what approaches might provide them with optimal comfort and reassurance. While this may see attitudes and therapeutic considerations shift away from our own reflexive inclinations, a platinum standard acknowledges that we cannot always be the perfect, infallible barometer of our patients' preferences, values, and goals.

The Platinum Rule also applies when guiding substitute decision makers. The question they must consider is not what they would want done, but what the patient would want done in this instance. *Imagine your critically ill dad six months ago and tell me what he would want us to do. Let's sit at his bedside and imagine saying "okay dad, you've been in hospital for two weeks. You've been unconscious for two days. The doctor says he doesn't think you are going to make it through the night, but he also thinks you have pneumonia, which in theory is treatable, but nobody knows how you're going to respond to that."*[6] The question is not what the substitute decision maker would want done, but what the father would want done *unto himself*—The Platinum Rule. This aligns with a substitute judgement standard,[8] wherein surrogates are asked to make decisions that patients would have made if they were competent. However, the Platinum Rule goes beyond simply trying to intuit what patients might want when they are unable to voice their wants and preferences, tapping into how all patients would wish to be perceived and treated. This requires confronting personal biases that might cause us to respond to patients according to our own ingrained perceptions and values— defaulting to a Golden standard—when nothing less than a Platinum standard will do.

Giving him the benefit of the doubt, one can easily imagine Bert's physician recommending MAiD from a position of wanting to mitigate current and future suffering. One can also easily imagine, based on the Golden Rule, that he offered a solution for a clinical situation he could neither fathom himself, or those he loved, being able to bear. Distorted compassion, however, represents a failure of the imagination. Perceptions of suffering can obstruct our ability to imagine patients experiencing life as having sustained meaning, purpose, and value, despite even overwhelming challenges. The Golden Rule has its place in medicine, given it provides an initial gauge in our response to patient suffering. But if we are truly intent on offering patient-centered care, consistent with *their* values, preferences and goals, consideration of the Platinum Rule is required: *doing unto patients as they would want done unto themselves.*

References

1. Personal communication, Dr. Cornelius Woelk, June 2021.
2. Marcelin JR, Siraj DS, Victor R, et al. The impact of unconscious bias in healthcare; how to recognize and mitigate it. *J Infect Dis.* 2019;220:S62–S73.
3. Frazee C. The vulnerable: who are they? https://www.virtualhospice.ca
4. Chochinov HM, McClement S, Hack T, et al. Eliciting personhood within clinical practice: effects on patients, families, and health care providers. *J Pain Symptom Manage.* 2015;49:974–980.
5. Kumagai AK, Lypson ML. Beyond cultural competence: critical consciousness, social justice, and multicultural education. *Acad Med.* 2009;84:782–787.
6. Personal communication, Dr. Mike Harlos, June 2021.
7. Phillips J, Wendler D. Clarifying substituted judgement: the endorsed life approach. *J Med Ethics.* 2015;41(9):723–730. doi: 10.1136/medethics-2013-101852. Epub 2014 Oct 30. PMID: 25360029.

13

Seeing Ellen and the Platinum Rule

Self-disclosure in caring for patients is not something I do casually. My rule of thumb is to reveal personal information only when it enhances or promotes the clinical work. Sharing personal information is a therapeutic strategy meant to serve the patient's purposes and address their needs, not the therapist's. For example, I might reveal my mother's or my sister's death to a patient struggling with grief, not for the sake of personal catharsis or to imply an equivalence to what they are going through, but to underscore that anyone who has had loving, meaningful connections is vulnerable to loss and this is an unavoidable and universal human experience. Sharing common ground can help patients feel less alone, better understood, and more hopeful they might eventually find their way.

I also tend to be restrained with self-disclosure in my publications. This piece about my sister Ellen is likely the most revealing I've been about my family and formative experiences. The truth is, I knew my sister Ellen as well as I've ever known another human being. I know with complete and utter certainty that Ellen would want her story told; that Ellen enjoyed being the focus of attention; and that Ellen would want her life to be the impetus for others to understand disability, vulnerability, and how overwhelming, frightening, and dismissive it feels not to be seen or acknowledged. That is why I chose to talk about this exquisitely private moment in her life in this piece called "Seeing Ellen and the Platinum Rule."

Seeing Ellen and the Platinum Rule. Harvey Max Chochinov. JAMA Neurology, 2022;79(11):1099. Reproduced with permission from *JAMA Neurology*. American Medical Association.

Several years before her death at the age of 55 years due to complications of cerebral palsy, my sister Ellen was again in hospital, this time in intensive care and on the brink of respiratory collapse and the possible need for intubation. To say cerebral palsy had shaped her life is an understatement, in that it molded nearly every facet of her being, from the contours of her body to the way she saw and experienced the world. And based on this, while one might assume that her life was defined by suffering, the only ones who suffered were those whose toes she managed to crush under the mighty weight of her electric wheelchair when she was on the dance floor.

With the passage of time, her body became increasingly contorted, affecting her ability to take a deep breath or fight off upper respiratory tract infections. So long as I can remember, blowing out birthday candles was impossible without the assistance of her nieces, nephews, friends, or extended family. Time at the family cottage in Winnipeg Beach, ice cream on a summer's day, chocolate milk, or meals prepared by my parents were among her greatest pleasures.

But health challenges often interfered with her various plans and wishful thinking that one day she might actually get to see the world. While being in hospital with Ellen was not an unfamiliar experience, this time felt different, with life and death hanging perilously in the balance. The attending physician, whom I knew from occasional work-related encounters, was diligently reviewing her medical record, scanning her monitors, and calculating if her deteriorating condition would soon require inserting a breathing tube.

At one point her physician turned to me, asking, "Does she read magazines"? While this was a seemingly innocent question, it was the only question I was asked about her personal life. The subtext was chilling, as this was not an attempt to get to know Ellen as a person or how she spent her days, but rather a cryptic way of deciding if hers was a life worth saving. While it was never said, I could intuit the rationale and detached mental calculus. Her body looks like a train wreck. Who would want to live this way? Perhaps we'd all be better off by letting nature take its course.

To be clear, this physician was not a bad person and was regarded as a highly skilled clinician. But the lens through which my sister was being viewed was one that had been shaped in ways her physician was entirely unaware of. From the time we are young, there are images and values that are elevated above all others, including youth, beauty, wealth, and power. We learn to worship at the altar of this ephemeral perfection, with all else deemed of lesser value, lesser utility, and lesser consequence. The results are insidious, from the way we perceive bodies—our own and those of others—to the social policies we do and do not support. It is no coincidence that older individuals, for instance, have been disproportionately affected by the COVID-19 pandemic, given our chronic failure to invest in the supports needed to safeguard their well-being and vitality. You bankroll what you value, and some lives are simply valued more than others.

But something else was happening that day at my sister's bedside that threatened to undermine the care she desperately wanted and needed. Treatment decisions are often based on considerations of reciprocity and The Golden Rule. If I were that patient, what would I want for myself? — doing unto others as we would want done unto ourselves. This means using our own values, wants, and needs as an indicator of those we assume are held by the patient. But what happens when these don't align? It is hard to imagine a wider chasm between my sister's lived experience and outlook, and that of her intensivist. When this degree of misalignment occurs, it is easy to anticipate health care recommendations based on the conviction that I wouldn't want to live that way. I wouldn't want to be that disabled, dependent, disfigured, or disenfranchised. Why offer opportunities to sustain an existence that I would personally find unimaginable and intolerable?

This is where a new standard of person-centered care—The Platinum Rule[1]—comes into play: *do unto others as they would want done unto themselves.* This means not presuming that we know what is in the patient's best interest based on what we would want in their circumstances and taking the time to consider what they would want, hope, or wish for. While not every patient request can be accommodated, The Platinum Rule provides insights that strip away biases and assumptions, helping us see who patients are as people and raising the bar on person-centered care. Not being seen erodes human dignity and undermines personhood, experiences that are at the core of human suffering.[2]

So when Ellen's physician asked me if she read magazines, I scrambled to come up with a response that would have this physician see beyond her distorted body and failing lungs. There wasn't enough time to talk about jiving on the dance floor or Winnipeg Beach or birthday celebrations.

I wanted Ellen to be seen as not just the patient, but the well-loved sister, daughter, aunt, niece, cousin, disability rights activist, and friend. I wanted everyone to understand that she had a rich emotional life, and an imagination that could take her to places that, as fate would have it, she would never get to see. And so, after a few seconds I responded, "Yes, she reads magazines. But only when she's in between novels."

References

1. Chochinov HM. The platinum rule: a new standard for person-centered care. *J Palliat Med.* 2022;25(6):854–856.
2. Cassel EJ. The nature of suffering and the goals of medicine. *N Engl J Med.* 1982;306(11):639–645.

14

Healthcare Provider as Witness

The story of Dr. Stuart Farber is one I've told countless times in presentations around the world. He used the metaphor of "my thread" to refer to his essence—how he saw himself as a person—and how that links with providing respectful care. Stuart was a colleague and a professor at the University of Washington Medical School, where he founded and directed the Palliative Care Service at the UW Medical Center. Sadly, he died too young but left behind important teachings and wisdom that continue to resonate.

Our paths first overlapped in the mid-1990s because of the Project on Death in America (PDIA). The PDIA was an initiative launched by the Open Society Institute in 1994. Its objective was to help transform the experience of dying in the United States by funding initiatives in professional and public education, the arts and humanities, research, clinical care, and public policy. Over the course of 9 years, PDIA distributed $45 million in grant awards to organizations and individuals working to improve care for dying patients and their families. Stuart was named a Soros Faculty Scholar by PDIA in 1995. I joined those ranks the following year, which is how we met.

The director of PDIA was Dr. Kathleen Foley. We'd first met in 1986, the year I started my fellowship at Memorial Sloan Kettering Cancer Center. At the time she was heading the country's first pain service in a cancer center and was the medical director of the Supportive Care Program. She was an unforgettable role model and teacher, who changed the way her trainees thought about what it meant to be a healthcare professional. She and her collaborator Nessa Coyle, a nurse practitioner and member of the Palliative Medicine Service at Memorial, helped shape me as a physician.

Shortly after receiving the PDIA scholarship, I recall meeting with Dr. Foley to discuss what this would mean for my future. The funding was meant to buy out my clinical time, freeing me up to take on various activities I'd outlined in my application (research, professional development, establishing multidisciplinary collaborations, etc.). During our

In Search of Dignity. Harvey Max Chochinov, Oxford University Press. © Oxford University Press 2025.
DOI: 10.1093/9780197805145.003.0014

conversation, I asked her, "What do you think is the most important thing I should be doing with all of this protected time?", to which she replied, "Harvey, you need to think."

At the time her response struck me as rather cryptic, even glib. But over the years I've come to appreciate the wisdom of those few, carefully selected words. Being a researcher and doing scholarly works requires time to think; time to consider big-picture issues or small irksome concerns and time to contemplate how to tackle seemingly unassailable problems. Doing this work has been the privilege of a lifetime, and I remain forever grateful to those who made this career path possible.

Healthcare Provider as Witness. Harvey Max Chochinov. *The Lancet*, 2016;388(10051):1272–1273. Reprinted with permission from Elsevier.

As he was approaching his own death, Stuart Farber, a palliative care physician, reflected on personhood and what he referred to as his thread: "With rare exception, the clinicians who treated me have good hearts, care deeply, but possess little or no knowledge of my thread. My thread is the narrative I use to make sense of my life. It is longitudinal, non-linear, emotional, filled with contradictions, and integrates my life experiences into a coherent whole. It is within the values and meanings of my story that treatment decisions are made. What contributes to meaning and quality is not about living longer but living a life that is consistent with my thread. Without knowing my thread, it is impossible for a clinician to provide respectful care."

So what does it mean to know a patient's "thread"? And why is it important that clinicians see their patients as persons, besides whatever ailment they happen to have? If, as Dr Farber suggests, how doctors see or perceive that thread determines our ability to deliver respectful care, we must reflect on the role of health-care provider as witness.

The word witness comes from the Old English *witnes*, meaning to attest to facts or events, based on personal knowledge; and is a literal translation of the Greek word *martyr*. In the Christian tradition, a martyr is someone who brings testimony, usually written or verbal, of their faith. As Christian testimonies were rejected and witnesses were put to death, the word martyr took on its contemporary meaning, referring to someone who suffers. Like witness, compassion implicates the notion of suffering and comes from the

Latin word *compati*, meaning to suffer with. For those who work in health care, being a witness is demanding and carries risks, for the observed and the observer alike.

Patients are under the ever-watchful gaze of health-care providers, making them vulnerable to our clinical perceptions. As witnesses, we must see and discern whatever ails our patients. Contemporary diagnostics allow us to probe the depths of the human body with great clarity and precision. And yet failure to see and acknowledge patients as whole persons can undermine their sense of intrinsic value and worth.

As he was facing advanced prostate cancer, the author Anatole Broyard wrote, "Just as he orders blood tests and bone scans of my body, I'd like my doctor to scan me, to grope for my spirit as well as my prostate. Without some such recognition, I am nothing but my illness . . . When a doctor refuses to acknowledge a patient, he is, in effect, abandoning him to his illness." Broyard yearns for a witness able to see not only his cancer, but also to recognize something essential regarding who he is as a person; perhaps, as Dr. Farber put it, his thread.

Patients need to recognize an affirming reflection of themselves in the eyes of those who care for them; a reflection that values personhood. If all they see reflected back is their problem checklist, probable diagnoses, and treatment options, they could feel that patienthood has eclipsed personhood. When patients recognize or sense, however, that their health-care provider acknowledges, or tries to acknowledge, what is genuinely important to them, dignity and personhood are likely to be upheld. Studies of dying patients by my research group have shown that over and above any symptoms or concerns we were able to measure, the most ardent predictor of sense of dignity is patients' perceptions of being seen—that is, being acknowledged and appreciated for who they are. Not being seen can feel like a repudiation of personhood.

What happens when the patient's thread is embedded within a fabric that is less recognizable to healthcare providers than Dr Farber's? What if, for instance, that fabric is woven from material that is shaped by disability or disenfranchisement or poverty? If someone securely placed within the social determinants of health must struggle to have personhood recognized, what chance does someone who is less securely positioned have to make themselves truly seen or known?

Catherine Frazee, a disabled Canadian educator, activist, and writer, has described the possible dangers of a myopic witness: "Having to wear diapers and drooling are highly stigmatized departures from what is expected of adult bodies. Those of us who deviate from these norms experience social shame and stigma that erodes resilience and increases vulnerability. The more deeply these stigmatized accounts are embedded in our discourse and social policy, the more deeply virulent social prejudice takes hold within our culture . . . What assurance can we offer that the physician who treats these adults at end-of-life will not stand at their bedside with horror—or revulsion—in his heart?"

A prejudicial witness in healthcare is a cause for concern. The word prejudice comes from the Latin *prae judicium*, meaning to inflict damage or judge in advance of knowing. Judging or making assumptions about patients without knowing their thread can cause great harm. Besides feeling devalued, disavowed, and discarded, patients may find themselves denied treatment options or guided toward others in ways that may not accord with their thread of values and desires; sometimes based on perceptions of suffering according to witnesses unable to genuinely see or acknowledge who patients really are.

The history of medicine is replete with examples of prejudice, usually based on the notion that unfamiliarity or "otherness" justifies an altered threshold for what constitutes ethical, moral, and compassionate practice. Between 1932 and 1972, the US Public Health Services studied rural African American men in Alabama without their informed consent, to determine the natural progression of untreated syphilis. Researchers knowingly failed to provide treatment, even after penicillin was validated as an effective cure. In the 1950s and 1960s, the Skid Row Cancer Study saw more than 1200 homeless men in Lower Manhattan have their prostates biopsied in exchange for promises of food and shelter, without being told of possible side-effects such as rectal tearing or impotence. Between the late 1950s and 1970s, children with intellectual disabilities at Willowbrooke State School were subject to experiments in which they were intentionally given hepatitis. The consequences of prejudice can be disastrous, which is why events like these often lead to tightening of regulations to protect participants in biomedical research. Being a skillful witness means being ever mindful of assumptions or biases that can influence how we perceive our patients, whether based on attitudes towards ageing, culture, race, religion, sexual orientation, gender, weight/size, socioeconomic class, or disability. These attitudes can distort our perceptions and lead us to bearing false witness.

What are the risks of being a witness? They include taking responsibility for pursuing an accurate diagnosis and formulating an effective treatment plan, knowing that all the while, the patient's health and wellbeing hang in the balance. In the hurly-burly of modern medicine, we tell ourselves that there is little time for anything else; and so, personhood falls off our clinical radar. But might restricting our vision to narrow clinical parameters mitigate a different kind of risk—the risk of feeling an emotional resonance with our patients' suffering? And yet not acknowledging personhood, along with disengagement and compartmentalization—"it's not my job"—are hallmarks of professional burnout. Being overwhelmed by our patients' suffering can render us ineffective, while only seeing the patient and not the person can eliminate the possibility of a genuine and compassionate response. So what is a capable witness to do?

Start by trying to know the patient's thread. Healthcare providers might consider asking patients, "what do I need to know about you as a person in order to give you the best care possible?" Our research group put that question to a group of critically ill patients; and their responses, contained within brief (less than 15 min) conversations, were instructive. Some shared that because of childhood trauma, they were afraid of authority figures "including people in white coats"; some said they were working hard to cover up that they were feeling confused; while others confessed to being afraid to die. Without exception, they wanted to convey some aspect of their story, with most indicating this information was important for their healthcare provider to know and that they believed it could improve their care. Healthcare providers who read these accounts in the clinical chart reported a heightened sense of respect and connection towards the patient; with openness to this information—in essence, seeing the patient's thread—being associated with their own job satisfaction. This suggests that being a compassionate witness requires generosity, humility, and the courage to look inward and acknowledge that the vulnerability we see is an affirmation of our own fragility and collective humanity. Furthermore, it affirms that broaching personhood yields important benefits for patients and healthcare providers alike.

Working in healthcare calls upon us to take on various tasks and assume many roles. As technology, medical innovation, and complex healthcare systems move us ever further away from the humanities of patient care, it is time we consider our duty, our responsibility, and our privilege to serve the role of witness.

15

Dying Well

Why We All Need to Have End-of-Life Conversations

My maternal great-grandmother Leah Litman was part of a Jewish organization of volunteers known as the Chevra Kadisha, tasked with preparing deceased Jews for burial. Their sacred obligation was to protect the body according to Jewish funeral tradition and, in accordance with Jewish law, to wash—but not embalm—it before placement in a plain burial shroud. My great-grandmother spent much of her time sewing those shrouds, traditionally white, simple, and pure linen. How all this shaped her feelings about death is hard to say. My now 94-year-old father remembers her taking him to the Jewish funeral home, years before she died, to show him the casket she'd chosen for herself. It would seem Leah Litman took death in her stride.

My grandfather Max (my middle name's sake) was cut out of similar cloth. He told my father that when his time came, we should plant grass and flowers around his grave and put up a bench so people could come visit.

Among the many things he did over the course of his successful and colorful career, my father was an insurance salesman. This meant dinner-table conversations that included how the cost of insurance premiums is based on the likelihood that someone would die. For some reason, this seemed perfectly normal and not the least bit upsetting. It certainly didn't dampen our appetites for my mother's wonderful cooking. Like his father Max Chochinov, my dad seems to have made peace with the idea of death.

Last year a dear friend confided in me that she and her husband didn't have wills. Being well into their seventh decade, this seemed inexplicable. When I asked her why, she told me that they just found the idea of thinking about death and planning for the possibility of death too upsetting. After explaining death wasn't a possibility but an inevitability, I walked her through why they needed wills and assured her that taking this action would neither hasten nor postpone death by a single moment. To this day, now having set her affairs in order, I occasionally begin our phone calls by sharing my delight she isn't dead yet.

In Search of Dignity. Harvey Max Chochinov, Oxford University Press. © Oxford University Press 2025.
DOI: 10.1093/9780197805145.003.0015

Not everyone is comfortable talking about death. But death is oblivious to our squeamishness and avoidance. Hence, end-of-life conversations are critical and necessary, and the best way to ensure your wishes and values inform whatever happens to you, when your time comes.

Dying Well: Why We All Need to Have End-of-Life Conversations by Harvey Max Chochinov. An earlier version of this essay first appeared in *Globe and Mail*, on April 14th, 2014.

The last time I was in Israel, I went on some home visits with a palliative care physician in the town of Sfat near the Sea of Galilee. My colleague, a devout Jewish doctor, took me to several homes to offer advice on managing his most serious, terminally ill patients. One older Chassidic Rabbi was dealing with an advanced lung cancer and having a difficult time accepting any kind of help from his young adult children. Next was a young Sephardic woman with advanced ovarian cancer, living in a small apartment with her mother and feeling abandoned by her other siblings. Then there was an elderly widow with far advanced breast cancer, struggling to get through her days because of poorly controlled pain.

In each encounter, the room would eventually fall silent, anticipating my response. To the ailing rabbi I said, "Children usually want to be with their parents when they are ill; it's a way of expressing that they care;" to the Sephardic young woman, I asked, "Do you think your brothers and sisters are keeping their distance because they are indifferent, or because they find it painful to see you so sick," and to the elderly woman I said, "You'll be feeling much better once your pain is under better control."

In each instance, nothing I said struck me as particularly profound, until, that is, I witnessed their responses. The rabbi shed a tear, thanked me and shook my hand. The Sephardic woman smiled as she let go some of her anger towards her brothers and sisters; and the elderly woman quickly retrieved a plastic bag, which she proceeded to fill with the various dried fruits and homemade pastries that bedecked her table and handed them over to me.

(Addendum: The other thing that made my trite comments more memorable was the fact that in each instance, my colleague would translate them into Hebrew. To me, Hebrew is the language of the Bible, the language of scriptures. I felt that the Hebrew version of my comments seemed to acquire

immediate spiritual heft—gravitas of biblical proportion—far beyond any-
thing they likely deserved. To my ear, in Hebrew, my pronouncements sounded
worthy of transcription on velum or parchment, or perhaps even stone tablets.
My colleague told me that for Israelis who speak only Hebrew, their experience
is exactly the opposite—that is, well-spoken English sounds scholarly, while
Hebrew, for them, sounds rather pedestrian.)

Teaching palliative care around the world, I am always struck by how similar people are, wherever they happen to live. In our humanity, we share very
common concerns and struggles regarding how to cope with vulnerability
and the inevitability of death.

Whenever my plane takes off, I always think about how air travel is the
perfect metaphor for life and death. The moment we are born, our lives take
flight. Some people remain airborne longer than others; some run into more
turbulence than others. Yet, most people are so engaged in the journey, they
ignore the fact that landings are inevitable. Working in palliative care, I can
assure you, there is a world of difference between a good and gentle landing,
as opposed to "crash and burn."

In our aversion to death, we are like the airline passenger who only wants
to think about the free food and complimentary drinks; check out what
movies are available, and periodically, look out the window and enjoy the
view. Focusing on the flight lets us shut out the reality that the ground we see
off in the far distance, is ground each one of us, without exception, must inevitably return to.

Not acknowledging death does not make it go away, any more so than
talking about it will somehow hasten its arrival.

Discussing death allows you to make plans and to make your wishes known
to loved ones. It allows you to state your preferences, affirm your values and
clarify your choices. Study after study indicates that it increases the likelihood that you will get the care you want, when you want it and where you
want it; and that it could spare your family the anguish of having to make
a decision on your behalf, should you no longer be able to communicate,
without knowing what you might have wanted under the circumstances.

These conversations do not have to wait until someone is dying. They can
happen anytime, given death is inescapable.

If all this sounds too daunting, here is some language you might want
to consider. Imagine turning to the person you have in mind and begin by
saying something like, "I love you." If that feels like a stretch, you can always
start with: "Look, I care about you, most of the time" or "What matters to

you matters to me." "When one of us gets sick or is facing the end, is there anything we should know about each other's wishes, to make sure we each get what we want?" You can also speak with your doctor and ask him or her about an advance directive and naming a healthcare proxy—that is, someone who will speak on your behalf when you are no longer able to do so for yourself.

Does that really sound so difficult? Do you really think that you are likely to hurt someone you love or care about by saying "I want to be able to make good choices for you, so tell me whatever you think I need to know to get it right."

After all, who doesn't want a gentle landing, as life itself comes to a complete and final stop.

16

In Search of a Good Death

My line of work makes me a magnet for discussions about death, dying, and loss. This happens pretty much anywhere and anytime—among friends and colleagues, in various social settings, sitting on an airplane, or standing in line to pay for groceries. Once people find out what I do professionally, these conversations are almost inevitable.

I recall once being driven from Edinburgh to Glasgow, where I was scheduled to speak at the Royal College of Physicians and Surgeons. My driver, who spoke with a very think Glaswegian accent, wanted to know what my lecture was about. I told him I planned to talk about palliative care, which (with his prompting) I explained was a part of medicine focused on advanced illness and end-of-life care. This unleashed an immediate and enthusiastic tirade I felt hard pressed to understand. He concluded by saying something that sounded like "What du ya thenk?" I assumed he wanted to talk about medical assistance in dying and responded by saying, "It's complicated, it's very complicated." It was clear to me, on this occasion, that dialect stood in the way of taking this conversation any further.

People usually want to tell me about their experiences of a loved one's illness, the struggles toward death, and the personal aftermath of loss and grief. Being taken into someone's confidence is humbling and revealing, given that it opens a window on how palliative care is being practiced and how it is evolving over time. I often come away from these encounters reassured that we are making progress, yet there are times I lament we haven't come far enough. At one shiva call, a grieving daughter described her mother's illness journey: when she'd initially become sick, some of the milestones of decline along the way, and various measures that had been put in place to navigate illness-related challenges. But the description of her mother's final hospitalization is one I will never forget. She told me about how much her mother had suffered, how overwhelming the pain had become, her "screaming," and the long hours of watching the clock between doses of medication. And then she said, "But the nurses were wonderful." I almost fell off my chair.

In Search of Dignity. Harvey Max Chochinov, Oxford University Press. © Oxford University Press 2025.
DOI: 10.1093/9780197805145.003.0016

There is nothing wonderful about inadequately controlled pain or health-care providers who don't provide patients impeccable symptom management as part of optimal, dignity-conserving palliative care. Since writing "In Search of a Good Death" 25 years ago, some progress has certainly been made. More people have access to palliative care, more medical schools and residency programs include specific training in palliative care, and slowly but surely there is increasing public awareness of palliative care. That said, we have a way to go. Each human being dies only once; we can't afford to get it wrong.

In Search of a Good Death by Harvey Max Chochinov. An earlier version of this essay first appeared in *Globe and Mail* on July 19th, 2000.

Imagine you're diagnosed with a terminal illness. If you're like most Canadians, your first response is, "Do I really want to think about this?" None of us like to ponder dying and its inevitability. Also, if you're like most Canadians, you probably assume that when your time comes, good end-of-life care will somehow accompany you as a matter of due course. But according to the report tabled last month by the Senate Social Affairs Subcommittee, *Quality End-of-Life Care: The Right of Every Canadian,* you'd better not count on it.

"In the five years since [the first Senate report] we have made little progress in the area of quality end-of-life care," Senator Sharon Carstairs, the Senate subcommittee chair, has said. "Canadians are still dying in needless pain and without adequate palliative care." Death itself seems indifferent to our lack of preparedness for its arrival. More than 220,000 Canadians die each year, 75 per cent of them in hospitals and long-term care facilities. But perhaps the most startling fact is that only an estimated 5 per cent will receive integrated, interdisciplinary palliative care—that is, care aimed at lessening physical, emotional, psychosocial, and spiritual suffering—rather than care that targets cure.

Since the Senate's last report, the number of institutional palliative-care beds across the country has actually fallen as result of health-care restructuring. Few provinces have designated palliative care as a core service with a specific budget.

I'm a psychiatrist and end-of-life-care researcher working in a Winnipeg palliative care unit. I am constantly in awe of my clinical colleagues and their incredible ability to alleviate pain and suffering in patients nearing death. I've often seen them sit at the bedside of someone in a pain crisis and not leave that patient's side until the crisis has passed. For them, attending to the dying is not an occasional or reluctantly undertaken task, and their successful management of patients' suffering is measured not in days of life endured, but rather quality of life lived. Their skill, knowledge and therapeutic effectiveness always leaves me feeling humbled. I know that suffering can often be diminished by appropriate care.

I recall one patient, a woman in her 40s with late stage cancer, who told us she wanted to die because of her unbearable pain. After our team managed to get her pain under control, she was able to live her last days at her family ranch, near her beloved horses. She told us about the intense joy of sitting on her back deck, drinking coffee and basking in sunlight. There are hundreds of similar stories; what's terrifying is so many others not like this.

What's the likelihood of getting this kind of expert care? How skilled are your health-care providers at managing symptoms of pain and discomfort? How aware are they of different therapeutic techniques, or of advances and multidisciplinary approaches?

According to the Senate report, there's no consistency in whether undergraduate medical students receive any palliative care education whatsoever. Few postgraduate medical programs have made palliative-care rotations mandatory. As for continuing medical education, there are some (largely underfunded) palliative-care programs, but the initiative to enroll in them is left to individual discretion. The Senate report urges that training and education of all professionals involved in end-of-life care should be made a priority.

Holes in the home-care safety net may force some terminally ill patients to check into hospital, where they may die in unfamiliar surroundings. We don't make home care easy enough. If someone you love is dying, and you need to take time away from work, do you have any assurances that your income will be protected, or that your job will remain secure in your absence? While provincial health plans pay for selected aspects of home-based palliative care, these plans don't always include the cost of drugs and equipment, such as pumps for pain medication, oxygen, and commodes. To care for patients at home, you may need private insurance, personal savings, or contributions from social agencies and service clubs to cover costs.

Women often shoulder the major portion of care, and make tremendous sacrifices to attend their dying parents, in-laws and siblings. But what we're asking of them is to be superhuman. We should support them by funding drug coverage, and professional and non-professional care services such as home nurses. Ottawa should offer income security and job protection for family members who care for the dying. We should have in place 24-hour pain-management teams and support for families, such as respite care and bereavement counselling.

Like every other area of medicine, developing good quality end-of-life care requires knowledge based on carefully conducted studies. Yet despite the fact we all die, there's a disturbing lack of research in Canada in this area, such as research into the effectiveness of medical and non-medical interventions and measures of appropriate, cost-effective, health-care services. We'll need to fund more research on dying if we want to make the best, most cost-effective decisions about care for the dying. And for their families.

Not long ago I worked with a terminally ill man who had clinical depression: What was the point of living another day? After treating his depression, he was able to enjoy his remaining days with his wife of 50 years. Good palliative care benefits not only patients, it has a ripple effect for those near to them.

Life is most vulnerable at its beginning and its ending. Sadly, the Senate report reads like an indictment of how little has been done to meet the needs of Canadians nearing death. Clearly, Ottawa and the provinces should act now to develop a national strategy for end-of-life care.

Yes, it may cost money, but as Senator Carstairs puts it, "As Canadians, we will afford what we value." We can't afford to ignore end-of-life care: Someday each of us will need it.

17

How People with Advanced Cancer Can Find Meaning Toward the End of Life

An Expert Perspective

I was asked to write this piece for CancerNet, which used to be the American Cancer Society's patient information portal until it was moved to Cancer. org. It was crafted for patients with terminal cancer. While it touches on important topics, such as meaning, reminiscence, legacy, and locating one's essence, it doesn't reflect how I normally speak with patients. Spending time with patients, especially those who are feeling vulnerable, is usually more about listening—carefully, sensitively, empathically—than it is about anything I might say. I certainly can't imagine delivering a monologue, including the one I've written below. That said, the piece is meant to be read, which means patients can choose when to read it, how much of it to read, and the pace that suits them best.

People feel anxious about what to say to someone who is suffering and vulnerable. I often hear, "I don't know what to say" or "I don't know the right thing to say." Embedded within those statements is an assumption that there is a right thing to say, or that there might be a special sequence of words that can make intolerable suffering tolerable. When someone dies, for instance, we might find ourselves searching for words to comfort to the bereft. Anxiety, desperation, and feelings of helplessness may result in us saying, "At least they aren't suffering," "It's God's will," "I suppose it was their time," and similar unhelpful, vacuous, hit-or-miss commiserations.

"I'm so sorry" is a much better place to start. Then shift your energy to listening, really taking in what the person has to say. Let them tell their story and express their anguish, anger, regret, remorse, and relief. They may raise questions or dilemmas, often rhetorical and unanswerable. This kind of listening gives people who are suffering a sense they are truly being heard, without judgment, and hence are being tenderly affirmed.

In Search of Dignity. Harvey Max Chochinov, Oxford University Press. © Oxford University Press 2025.
DOI: 10.1093/9780197805145.003.0017

I recall being asked to see the wife of a man with end-stage gastrointestinal cancer who was nearing his final days. She was reticent to involve palliative care, despite his hospital care team's struggle to get him comfortable. Late one evening, while the physician on call was reevaluating the situation, I asked if she'd like to go for a walk with me. We entered the elevator and, with her permission, we headed up to the eighth floor, which houses our palliative care unit. As we stepped onto the ward, few words passed between us. The lighting was muted; there was a sense of calm as the only sounds were those scattered conversations between patients and their visitors drifting into the hallway. We made our way to the glass atrium at the end of the hallway overlooking the city, turned around, and made our way back. As we entered the elevator, she turned to me and said, "I get it."

Words are important, and I hope patients choosing to read this article find comfort and reassurance. That said, we must be mindful that silence can be golden.

How People with Advanced Cancer Can Find Meaning Toward the End of Life: An Expert Perspective by Harvey Max Chochinov. An earlier version of this essay first appeared on CancerNet in 2023.

Let me begin by saying that if you have received an end-stage cancer diagnosis and whatever you are doing to cope is comfortable for you, just keep doing it. But if it isn't working as well as you'd like, here are some thoughts for you to consider.

First, I wish I had the words to take away your anguish or fundamentally change what is happening to you. Like a beautiful piece of music, a stirring play, or an engrossing book, endings almost always leave us longing for one more chorus, one more act, or one more chapter. That is how we humans are wired.

The details of when and how your life is coming to an end will likely color and shape your feelings of sadness, longing, and grief. This is perfectly natural. Like other losses you may have experienced throughout your life, you know these feelings are unavoidable. You need to give yourself permission to experience these emotions rather than searching for what may be ineffective ways of avoiding them, such as prohibiting conversations that trigger sadness, use of alcohol, or isolation.

Your difficult feelings mean that what is ending was important to you and that you were connected and engaged, either with people, ideas, responsibilities, roles, an identity, or a purpose. In other words, despite its challenges, your life mattered to you. And for humans, meaning is like oxygen; we simply can't live without it.

As your life draws to a close, you may struggle with how to carry on when so many of the things that give you meaning are slowly being taken away. And how do you somehow sustain meaning to live out your final days, until time eventually runs out? Although there is no "one size fits all" response, here are some things for you to think about.

1: Meaning can come through reminiscence.

Approaching the end of life—whether you have days, weeks, months, or a year or 2 left—is the only time your entire life story, from start to finish, is available to you. Some people find meaning through the process of reminiscence. This allows them to integrate the pieces that have shaped their lives and, perhaps for the first time, see how these pieces make sense within the fullness of their completed life. Like music, theatre, or literature, endings matter and shape the way we understand or appreciate the experience in its entirety. This kind of integration and broad life perspective might protect you from feelings of despair.

2: Remember that your life matters.

You may find yourself wondering whether your life mattered as you approach its end. It is worth remembering that never in the entirety of human existence has there been, nor will there ever be, another person exactly like you. However you see yourself, there is no denying the uniqueness of you. This may lead you to contemplate the importance of legacy and what of yourself you want left behind. Attending to your legacy can offer meaning and comfort for you and your family, even towards the end of life.

For some people, legacy is about expressions of love, regret, and forgiveness shared with those who matter. These words or conversations can generate memories that will extend beyond death and reside in the collective memories of those left behind. For some people, this is a time to share stories and memories, bestow insights or wisdom, express hopes and wishes, and offer guidance for those you care about. Dignity therapy is one way people anticipating the end of life can engage in these important, meaningful conversations. During Dignity Therapy, the therapist makes a written record of the conversation for the person to give to those they wish to carry their memory into the future. Talk with your health care team about what therapy services may be available to you.

3: Try to separate what approaching death can take away from you and what remains within your grasp that can help you sustain meaning.

Living with a life-limiting illness like advanced cancer can challenge your ability to do many things. But the ultimate challenge, especially in the face of no longer being able to do those things, is your capacity to hold onto the essence of who you are.

What does it mean to be you when you can no longer do the things that were part of being you? Meaning often arrives by way of connecting with your essence or core as a person. Until you lose consciousness, which generally happens towards the very end of life, people usually maintain their ability to convey their thoughts or feelings. They can still embody the presence that is the uniqueness of who they are and the place they hold in the lives of those who care about them and those they are connected to.

Some people may also take comfort in knowing that, even towards the end of life, they are giving those who care about them an opportunity to follow a path of least regret. Every experience, conversation, disclosure, or time shared together with loved ones creates lasting memories and shapes the grief that will soon follow. Even when words are no longer possible, your presence offers those within your circle a place to gather and begin mourning; a place to comfort and support one another as they contemplate how to move forward in their lives without you. Whatever your final path towards death, know that it will imprint those who grieve your passing and how they face the end when their time comes. That is something you will shape until you take your final breath.

18

Health Care, Health Caring, and the Culture of Medicine

Ten years ago, I wrote this article introducing the term "health caring." Too often our healthcare system focuses on transactional medicine while overlooking relational considerations (see Chapters 24 and 26). Health caring insists on both. While I still find the idea compelling, it hasn't taken hold the way I hoped it might. Since then, I've come to appreciate how the tail of knowledge translation can be incredibly long. It can take years, even decades for an idea to get the traction it needs to make a real difference. Shortening that tail takes concerted effort and is what knowledge translation and implementation science are all about.

As a young researcher, I didn't given this much thought. I assumed once a study was complete and published, knowledge dissemination would happen as a matter of due course; that is, I imagined my papers would find their way into the hands of clinicians, hence transforming practice. I recall organizing a coffee-and-donut gathering at the hospital where we'd recruited patients for a recently completed study. I saw to it that copies of the article were on hand for those wanting to learn more about our findings. As the event was winding down, my wonderful research nurse Beverly took me aside and said, "Harvey, you know no one ever reads your papers!" It was a hilarious moment of epiphany. Bev was not implying that the research was unimportant, or that the publication didn't matter; she was simply saying that that is not enough. And she was right.

Dignity Therapy is an example of successful knowledge translation. While the original paper on Dignity Therapy appeared in the Journal of Clinical Oncology *in 2005, it has taken nearly 20 years of concerted effort to move this novel psychotherapeutic intervention into mainstream practice. My book* Dignity Therapy: Final Words for Final Days *has now been translated into German, Portuguese, Italian, Hungarian, Chinese, Japanese, and Korean. Over the past two decades, I have given hundreds of lectures worldwide, explaining how Dignity Therapy came into being, how*

In Search of Dignity. Harvey Max Chochinov, Oxford University Press. © Oxford University Press 2025.
DOI: 10.1093/9780197805145.003.0018

it is administered, and its empirical basis. There are now over 100 empirical papers and about a dozen systematic reviews, attesting to the utility and efficacy of Dignity Therapy in various clinical settings. Since its inception, it has spread from palliative care to other vulnerable populations, including patients with earlier stages of malignancy, those with neurodegenerative disorders, the seriously mental ill, patients with early to moderate dementia, and the frail elderly. I have conducted scores of international workshops on Dignity Therapy, and other such training is being offered by colleagues who have embraced Dignity Therapy in various countries around the world. Over the past 20 years, Dignity Therapy has been referenced in most major textbooks on palliative care, geriatric medicine, and psychological care for the terminally ill. It has also been profiled in various newspapers in the United States, including The Washington Post, *along with Canada, Australia, New Zealand, and Brazil.*

The way Dignity Therapy has taken hold illustrates how knowledge translation extends the reach of clinical innovation. The idea of health caring isn't there yet. Perhaps over time, with some concerted effort to spread the word, health caring may get the traction it needs, helping shift the arc of medicine toward kindness, empathy, and compassion.

Health Care, Health Caring, and the Culture of Medicine. Harvey Max Chochinov. *Current Oncology.* 2014; 21(5):668–669. Reuse granted under CC BY license.

At first glance, "care" and "caring" hardly seem distinguishable. Add health into the mix, however, and the differences are striking. We readily speak about a system of "health care," but no one talks about "health caring." The former refers to the delivery of evidence-based medicine and how it can be provided in a fashion that is efficient, equitable (this being a Canadian perspective), and cost-effective. Health care is designed to provide for the medical needs of patients—a designation primarily based on the specifics of a diagnosis and treatment.

However, despite its considerable merits, health care can sometimes be emotionally abrasive or harsh. No one wants to be seen just in terms of their ailment or to have their needs reduced to little more than a treatment algorithm—which is why no one likes to be a patient. Being a patient means having to yield to the whims of a medical condition and to bend to the regulations and rigidities of the health care system. The word "patient" comes from the same Latin derivative as "patience." Clearly, it takes great patience to be a patient, and the sicker a person is, the more that patience is put to the test.

Over and above an illness or concern, health care pushes people further into patienthood. That push can be as subtle as a plastic identification bracelet, as annoying as being kept waiting to be seen, as demoralizing as thoughtless violations of privacy; and even occasionally assaultive, wherein patienthood seems to eclipse personhood entirely.

Mrs. J was a 47-year-old woman, mother of three teenagers, with metastatic breast cancer. Despite the various complications of her illness and treatment, she had managed to cope relatively well. However, that changed when, during the process of simulation, her radiation oncologist failed to warn her that he would be using a felt pen to mark her treatment fields on her chest wall. Without knowing why the marking was happening, she felt "like a slab of meat," "a piece of paper." She was so distraught that she considered withdrawing from treatment altogether, and she remained distrustful and frightened throughout her ensuing course of radiation therapy.

To be sure, Mrs. J's management was technically accurate, and evidence based. Little doubt that it was also carried out with the best of intentions, designed to guide the delivery of optimal radiation to mitigate the effects of her progressive breast cancer. Her experience, however, typifies the point at which health care often fails to realize its full and humane potential, the potential of "health caring."

If health care is designed to address the needs of patients, health caring is ever mindful that patients are people with feelings that matter. Those feelings almost always include a heightened sense of vulnerability, dependency, and loss of control, which can be internally driven by the underlying condition, but also externally imposed (depending on the quality and tone of the health care encounter), resulting in threatened self-efficacy and personhood.

Health caring must always ask the questions "How might this make a person feel" or "How does it feel to be kept waiting, examined, drawn on," or questions addressing the multitude of experiences that patients are asked to endure. Asking the question shifts the frame of reference, changing the way in which clinicians perceive and respond to patients. It also shifts the care tenor—that is, the emotional and empathic qualities of a clinical encounter as shaped by the health care provider. Health caring insists that attending to the needs of the patient goes hand-in-hand with sensitivity to the feelings of the person. To be sure, that approach will not eliminate the toils of patienthood (case in point, radiation fields still need to be marked). But applying the lens of health caring—"How might this make a person feel?"—changes the tone of care, eliciting clear explanations, perhaps a gentle touch, a kind word, or an understanding look. Those are ways of acknowledging personhood, and they are critical elements of our clinical repertoire.

Finally, although the term "patient" is generic and applies to a broad clinical designation, the term "person" denotes completely opposite qualities. "Person" and "individual" are synonymous. Knowing someone means having some understanding of who they are as a unique individual. Where health care asks about a problem, health caring asks "What do I need to know about you as a person to give you the best care possible?" Those questions are not mutually exclusive, and yet one without the other is simply not good enough. Health caring elicits trust, fuller patient disclosure, and accurate assessment of the goals of care. It heightens patient satisfaction and decreases the likelihood of complaints or litigation. Health caring might even enhance job satisfaction. By putting personhood on the clinical radar, health care providers can reconnect with core values that likely attracted them into their work in the first place. Realizing the differences between "health care" and "health caring" could go a long way in transforming the culture of medicine.

19

Intensive Caring

Reminding Patients They Matter

On May 22, 2023, I had the honor of delivering the Cicely Saunders International Lecture. The organizers describe this lectureship as "an annual event hosted by the Cicely Saunders Institute, King's College London." It is designed to feature the work of speakers who are "global leaders, whose work has significantly influenced the field" and offers a unique opportunity "to learn from world-leading clinicians and scientists, aimed at clinicians, healthcare researchers, health policymakers and palliative care funders."

The topic of my lecture, "Intensive Caring: Reminding Patients They Matter," was inspired by Dame Cicely Saunders, who founded the modern hospice movement. My connection with Dame Cicely and St. Christopher's Hospice traces back to my nearly 30-year friendship with Dr. Irene Higginson. Dr. Higginson is currently the Executive Dean of the Faculty of Nursing, Midwifery & Palliative Care and is Professor of Palliative Care & Policy at King's College London. She is the Founding Professor of the Cicely Saunders Institute, Honorary Consultant in Palliative Medicine, National Institute for Health and Care Research Emeritus Senior Investigator, and Fellow of the Academy of Sciences. She is in the top 1% of highly cited researchers in the world and in 2008 was named to the Order of the British Empire for services to medicine.

When we first met at a meeting in Banff, Alberta, sometime in the mid-1990s, she was simply "Irene from London"—a young, dynamic palliative care physician and researcher whose reputation I was only coming to appreciate. She was generous with her mentorship and guidance and in 2002 invited me to speak at King's College and to meet, for the first time, Dame Cicely Saunders.

Dame Cicely is to palliative care what Mick Jagger is to rock and roll. As the date of my talk drew nearer, April of that year as I recall, my anxiety began to mount. Dame Cicely had an extraordinary reputation for her pioneering work in palliative care but was known to be intellectually exacting

In Search of Dignity. Harvey Max Chochinov, Oxford University Press. © Oxford University Press 2025.
DOI: 10.1093/9780197805145.003.0019

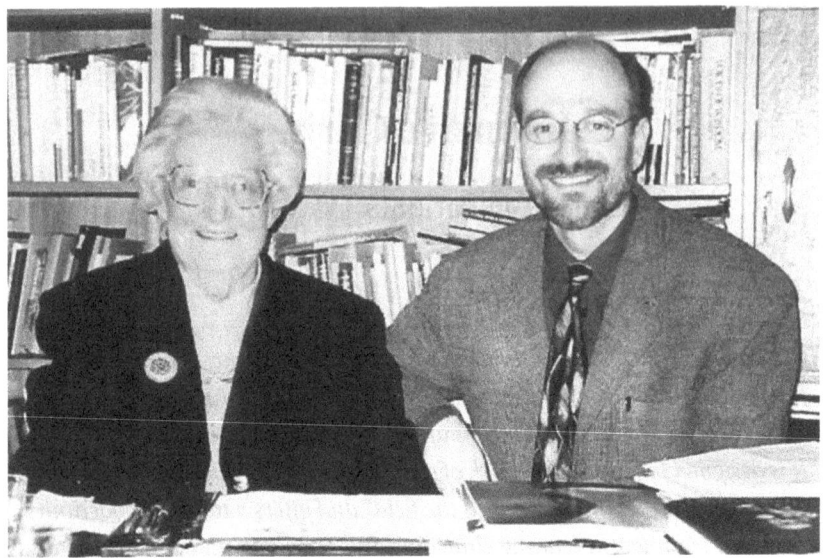

Figure 19.1 The author with Dame Cicely Saunders

and didn't suffer fools gladly. As my departure date for London approached, I began reviewing my research papers, anticipating being grilled within an inch of my life.

The morning of my talk, I hailed a taxi from my hotel near St. Pancras Station and asked to be taken to St. Christopher's Hospice. My anxiety held fast when the driver said, "Of course, everyone knows who Dame Cicely Saunders is!" Upon my arrival, I was shown into a rather formal, austere waiting room, where I was to remain until the appointed meeting time. I'll never forget the feeling of foreboding as a voice came booming over the intercom, announcing, "The Dame will see you now." I walked in, and Irene made introductions and snapped a photograph (Figure 19.1).

As it happens, Dame Cicely did not ask me a single question about my work. Truth be told, I'm not sure she'd ever heard of me before I walked into her study that day. She did, however, ask me one question: "Would you care for a sherry?" She reached back into a cupboard on the right side of her bookshelf, pulled out two glasses (seen in lower left corner of the picture), and poured two stiff drinks. It was 10 a.m., just before I was to give a lecture for the students and faculty of the King's College Department of Palliative Care. But she was Dame Cicely Saunders; and when Dame Cicely asks, "Would you care for a sherry?" there is only one answer. And that answer is "yes."

Intensive Caring: Reminding Patients They Matter. Harvey Max Chochinov. *Journal of Clinical Oncology*, 2023;41(16):2884–2887. Reprinted with permission from Wolters Kluwer Health Inc.

Introduction

Dame Cicely Saunders, the founder of the modern hospice movement and palliative care, famously said, *You matter because you are you, and you matter to the last moment of your life.*[1] This quote is the central philosophical tenet of palliative care. It implores us to remind patients, who may be feeling helpless, hopeless, or worthless, that *they matter.* Even when they feel life is no longer worth living, we, their healthcare professionals, must affirm their intrinsic worth, for all that they are, all that they were and all that they will become in the collective memories of those they will eventually leave behind. While Dame Cicely gave us this inspiring direction, missing is a well-articulated approach centered on affirming patients matter. This approach, which I will coin *Intensive Caring,* incorporates various empirically derived components that collectively describe a way of being with patients who have lost hope, who have lost any sense of meaning or purpose, and who ultimately feel they *no longer matter.*

Why It Matters to Matter

There is abundant evidence that patients approaching death are susceptible to feeling they *no longer matter.* Our own research demonstrates that patients approaching death may feel a burden to others;[2] that life is futile and an affliction to those they feel incumbered by having to look after them. Self-perceived burden is contagious and self-perpetuating; patients who experience it may cause family members to feel helpless and exhausted, tacitly affirming that they are indeed a burden.[3] Feeling a burden has consistently been reported as a driver of desire for death, loss of will to live, and interest in physician-hastened death.[3] From the patient's perspective, death offers a way to relieve the burden they sense they have become, while ending a life they feel *no longer matters.*

I recall one such patient early in my career, who struggled with feelings of futility and hopelessness in the face of end-stage brain cancer. He'd been admitted to an inpatient neuro-oncology ward, where he felt a burden to his healthcare team and wanted me to help him die. He saw little point in continuing his life, which had been marked by bipolar disorder, polysubstance abuse, and family estrangement; he emphatically felt he no longer mattered. I told him that I could not and would not hasten his death, but was prepared to support him in any way that I could until the very end. We began to meet weekly, occasionally twice a week, while I delved into learning more about who he was, including the origins of his chronic self-loathing. He would often complain about things such as hospital routines, the medical staff—and one day began to berate me and the futility of my efforts to help him. Being young and naïve, I suggested that if our meetings were not helpful, neither of us were under any obligation to continue. He responded as if I'd gone mad. "Are you crazy?" he said. "These appointments are the only thing that keep me going!"

Elements of Intensive Caring

Intensive Caring requires finding ways to remind patients they still matter (Table 19.1). A foundational element of this approach is **nonabandonment**, which demands committed, ongoing care and caring, even when patients no longer care about themselves. Dame Cicely wrote "suffering is only intolerable when nobody cares."[1] Absent someone who cares, suffering, like cancer, can grow, spread, and even kill. Studies have shown that when patients feel abandoned and bereft of care, they are more likely to contemplate or to die by suicide.[4] Other studies have reported that a sustained, quality connection between patients and their oncologist provides better protection against suicidal ideation than mental health interventions, including psychotropic medications.[5] Our studies on desire for death in the terminally ill found those who desire death report lower family support relative to those who don't.[6] Hence, the assurance of continued caring and support is a vital component of helping patients feel *they matter.*

Table 19.1. Elements of Intensive Caring

- Nonabandonment[4,5,6]
  - Committed, quality connection
  - Ongoing support
- Taking an interest in the patient as a person[7,8,9]
  - Enhance empathy, respect, connectedness
  - Affirm worth of who they are, were, or tried to be and what they achieved or tried to accomplish
- Knowing What is Possible: Holding/containing hope[10-15]
  - Finding hope for psychological, spiritual, and physical comfort
  - Hope for minimal suffering and a peaceful death
  - Finding meaning and purpose in
    - Relationships
    - Imparting words/sentiments that need to be shared, such as reconciliation, forgiveness, love, affirmation of feelings
    - Modeling how to die
  - Guiding families toward viable opportunities[15]
    - 5 Time
    - Connection
    - Comfort
    - Forgiveness
    - Goodbyes
- Dignity affirming tone of care/therapeutic presence[16]
  - Being compassionate and empathic
  - Being respectful and nonjudgmental
  - Being genuine and authentic
  - Being trustworthy
  - Being fully present
  - Valuing intrinsic worth of the patient
  - Being mindful of boundaries and being emotionally resilient
- Therapeutic humility[16]
  - Tolerate clinical ambiguity
  - Accept and honor the patient's expertise
  - Trust in the process
  - Avoid the need to fix.

Another component of *Intrinsic Caring* is **taking a keen interest in who the patient is as a person.** Our studies of the Patient Dignity Question (PDQ), which asks "what do I need to know about you as a person to give you the best care possible," helps patients feel they are seen as whole persons, rather than the embodiment of their disease or disability.[7] A recent study of more than 2,000 inpatients and outpatients being seen at a quaternary care cancer center in the USA reported that the PDQ can be used as a means of eliciting values among patients with advanced malignancies.[8] Being appreciated in this holistic way helps safeguard patients' dignity.

Acknowledging personhood must follow principles of unconditional positive regard, conveying appreciation for who they are, what they are, and all they've tried to be.[9] It also enhances healthcare professionals' connectedness, respect, and empathy toward patients, establishing that besides the particulars of their clinical status, who they are as a person matters.[7]

When patients feel they *don't matter*, hopelessness is never far afield. Studies consistently show a strong connection between hopelessness and suicidality.[10,11] Our own palliative care research affirms that hopelessness is a strong predictor of desire for death.[10] *Intensive Caring* sees healthcare professionals **know what is possible and hold or contain hope** when patients can no longer do so themselves. This means expanding one's therapeutic imagination to include the possibility that patients may find psychological, spiritual, and physical comfort, tolerable suffering and for those near the end, a peaceful death. Toward end of life, hope tends to conflate with meaning and purpose, and may be nurtured through connections to those who, or things that, matter. This may include affirming that all that needs saying has been said, or bears repeating. Studies have shown that clinical approaches that facilitate sharing this kind of information mitigate psychological distress, enhance end-of-life experience,[12,13] and provide families comfort.[14] Healthcare professionals can also guide families along a path marked by opportunities for connection, comfort, forgiveness, and goodbyes.[15]

Patients may also find meaning or take comfort in knowing they are preparing loved ones they will soon leave behind. I recall a young woman with metastatic breast cancer who, in the context of dignity therapy,[12] offered wisdom to help guide her infant daughter into the future, shared reminiscences to help her family sustain the memory of her all too short life; thanked her parents and siblings for the love and support that had shaped who she was as a person, and gave her husband permission to find happiness, including a new partner, as he moved forward into a life without her. These kinds of opportunities extend to the very end of life. As Dame Cicely said, "How people die remains in the memory of those who live on."[1] For some, meaning and purpose may reside in knowing that in their dying, they will have provided a template for how one leaves this precious life.

Intensive Caring requires **a tone of care that is dignity affirming.** We have studied this tone, which we labeled Therapeutic Presence.[16] The latter comprises being compassionate and empathic, being respectful and non-judgmental, being genuine and authentic, being trustworthy, being fully present, valuing the intrinsic worth of the patient, being mindful of boundaries, and being emotionally resilient. Cumulatively, this tone of care, independent of words or actions, affirms patients' worth, provides the respect they deserve, while affirming they genuinely matter.

The Need for Therapeutic Humility

Intensive Caring requires **therapeutic humility**. The standard medical paradigm—examine, diagnose, and fix—is empowering, but within the realm of human suffering, some problems simply defy repair. Therapeutic humility means relinquishing the need to *fix*, along with tolerating clinical ambiguity, accepting and honoring the patient as expert, and trusting in the process.[16] There are cancers that can't be cured, depressions that resist treatment, and suffering whose intensity seems impenetrable. In those instances, the goal to *fix* can lead to feelings of failure and an inclination to withdraw. Colluding with the patient's hopelessness can find healthcare professionals affirming that indeed, all is futile and life itself, inconsequential. Ironically, while this may heighten a sense of mutual understanding and even connectedness, it is a therapeutic dead end, with death the only apparent way to fix patients' suffering. Therapeutic humility sees notions of *fixing* yield to commitment to understand the nature of the patient's suffering, while creating a safe space to bear witness, to validate, and to comfort always. Healthcare professionals must also appreciate the therapeutic potency of having patients express their suffering, while acknowledging their experience, thus lightening their load and decreasing their sense of isolation.

Tolerating ambiguity is not easy as it means walking a clinical path fraught with uncertainty, in the absence of our usual therapeutic tools aimed at *fixing*. Collegial support can help sustain us through this kind of work. *Intensive Caring* can be especially taxing when caring for those teetering between life and death and applies, whether patients are living with advanced cancers, or struggling with conditions where death is not reasonably foreseeable. For many years, I cared for one such woman, whose successful academic career unraveled after cancer surgery left her with chronic pain, leading to intense residual depression. Years of myriad treatments, hospitalizations, and ECT were unable to help her reclaim the essence of who she once was. When she felt close to the edge, I'd remind her that our work together *mattered, that she mattered,* and that I remained committed to seeing her. At times it seemed our steadfast connection was the only thing keeping her tethered to life. One day, 2 weeks after introducing yet another (this time newly released) anti-depressant, she sat down in her chair, turned to me, and declared "the office door is purple." I pointed out that it had always been purple, to which she gleefully replied, "I know, but now I care!" Continued involvement offers the opportunity to sustain patients and sometimes, even the potential for healing.

Conclusion

Intensive Caring, the therapeutic derivative of Dame Cicely's "You matter because you are you," provides a way of being with patients who have come to believe their lives are no longer of any consequence. Just as Intensive Care was designed to address the needs of patients with severe and life-threatening conditions, *Intensive Caring* offers a way for *all* healthcare professionals to be with patients confronting the enormity of human suffering. While trying to fix what is intrinsically broken can leave healthcare professionals feeling helpless and like they are failing, *Intensive Caring* provides an opportunity to target achievable goals, focused on myriad ways of affirming that patients matter. Its individual elements are well described in the literature and collectively encompass presence, compassion, and hope. While cross cultural resonance of *Intensive Caring* remains to be seen, the notion of personhood and the need to feel one matters is universal and speaks to the essence of what it is to be human. It has been more than 50 years since Dame Cicely shared the wisdom informing this clinical approach. Decades later, when medicine's reach *to fix* exceeds its grasp, the time to consider the role of *Intensive Caring* is now.

References

1. Cicely Saunders quotes: https://www.azquotes.com/author/20332-Cicely_Saunders.
2. Chochinov HM, Kristjanson LJ, Hack TF, et al. Burden to others and the terminally ill. *J Pain Symptom Manage.* 2007;34:463–471.
3. McPherson CJ, Wilson KG, Murray MA. Feeling like a burden to others: a systematic review focusing on the end of life. *Palliat Med.* 2007;21:115–128.
4. Allebeck P, Bolund C. Suicides and suicide attempts in cancer patients. *Psychol Med.* 1991;21:979–984.
5. Trevino KM, Abbott CH, Fisch MJ, et al. Patient-oncologist alliance as protection against suicidal ideation in young adults with advanced cancer. *Cancer.* 2014;120:2272–2281.
6. Chochinov HM, Wilson KG, Enns M, et al. Desire for death in the terminally ill. *Am J Psychiatry.* 1995;152:1185–1191.

7. Chochinov HM, McClement S, Hack T, et al. Eliciting personhood within clinical practice: effects on patients, families, and health care providers. *J Pain Symptom Manage.* 2015;4:974–980.

8. Hadler RA, Goldshore M, Rosa WE, Nelson J. "What do I need to know about you?": the Patient Dignity Question, age, and proximity to death among patients with cancer. *Support Care Cancer.* 2022;30:5175–5186.

9. Rogers CR. *Client-Centered Therapy: Its Current Practice, Implications and Theory.* Houghton Mifflin; 1951.

10. Chochinov HM, Wilson KG, Enns M, Lander S. Depression, hopelessness, and suicidal ideation in the terminally ill. *Psychosomatics.* 1998;39:366–370.

11. Breitbart W, Rosenfeld B, Pessin H, et al. Depression, hopelessness, and desire for hastened death in terminally ill patients with cancer. *JAMA.* 2000;284:2907–2911.

12. Chochinov HM. *Dignity Therapy: The Human Side of Medicine.* Oxford University Press; 2011.

13. Breitbart W, Poppito SR. *Meaning-Centered Group Psychotherapy for Patients with Advanced Cancer: A Treatment Manual.* Oxford University Press; 2014.

14. McClement S, Chochinov HM, Hack T, et al. Dignity therapy: family member perspectives. *J Palliat Med.* 2007;10:1076–1082.

15. Kristjanson LJ, Aoun S. Palliative care for families: remembering the hidden patients. *Can J Psychiatry.* 2004;49:359–365.

16. Chochinov HM, McClement SE, Hack TF, et al. Health care provider communication: an empirical model of therapeutic effectiveness. *Cancer.* 2013;119:1706–1713.

20

Intensive Caring

Reminding Families They Matter

---

*The two articles on Intensive Caring (in this chapter and the previous one)
take on the question of how to respond to patients when cure or fix is not
possible. While most people are familiar with the maxim "To cure sometimes, to relieve often, to comfort always," it lacks sufficient direction in
how to attend to someone whose health circumstances are intractable or
incurable. In palliative care, our clinical efforts are focused on quality of
life, the enhancement of comfort, and the amelioration of symptoms despite
advancing, life-limiting illness. That said, a taxonomy for how to be with or
address suffering—described in these two chapters on Intensive Caring—
offers guidance to those entering this clinically challenging space.*

*The idea of "things that can't be cured" was something I grew up with. My
sister, Ellen Chochinov, lived with significant disabilities (see* Chapter 13*).
In our home, disability wasn't a problem to be solved—no more so than
the number of hours in a day—but something that was part of our lives.
Although it's been 16 years since she died, my reflections on her life are well
captured in her obituary, published in the* Globe and Mail *on December
17, 2009.*

Ellen Chochinov's entrance into this world was not an easy one. Born with
cerebral palsy, she worked hard not to let it define her life even though it
shaped her body. Ellen was the oldest of three children of Dave and Shirley
Chochinov. Despite being told it was futile, my mother taught Ellen to
read. Family members joked that for a book or movie to be rated "E" for
Ellen, it had to include heavy doses of romance, medical drama, tragedy
and dollops of sap—the more sap the better. Growing up with Ellen meant
learning to count the number of stairs at each entrance, check the height

In Search of Dignity. Harvey Max Chochinov, Oxford University Press. © Oxford University Press 2025.
DOI: 10.1093/9780197805145.003.0020

of tabletops, notice the presence or absence of a bevelled curb or the width of a corridor and take note of the number of buttons, zippers and snaps on a piece of clothing. In later years, added to the list was the consistency of foods—what could be easily swallowed and what might induce choking.

Knowing Ellen meant seeing the world through a different lens, a lens that acknowledged differences and tried to accommodate them rather than pretending we live in a world of uniform shapes and capacities. Ellen was an enigma. At times she was impossible to please. On other occasions, her happiness was as straightforward as an easy smile and a gentle touch. She loved an attentive listener, seeing a movie, a family gathering and a day or weekend at her beloved Winnipeg Beach. These could dull the pain, distract her from her problems and satisfy her completely. She loved to have fun and loved anyone who loved her in return. Given her electric wheelchair, music and a dance floor, we sometimes wondered if she didn't take wicked pleasure in crushing as many toes or bruising as many ankles as possible.

They say it takes a village to raise a child. Given Ellen's immobility, my parents and extended family did everything possible to make that village feel like an entire universe. Every birthday, anniversary, holiday, any pretense whatsoever to gather and celebrate, helped make Ellen feel that "if this is my village, the circus is almost always in town."

Ellen cared deeply about disability rights and wasn't shy to raise her voice. If there is a heaven, it is a place where Ellen's effortless laughter can be heard. Somewhere off in the distance, her wheelchair is tumbling down a bottomless abyss as she dances carefree, supported by her strong and perfectly shaped legs for the first time. Her life should remind us to be tolerant of one another, to treat each other with kindness and respect, and to be united by our humanity rather than divided by what sets us apart. We hope to pass that along to our children and they to their children. In that way, Ellen's memory and legacy will live on.

Intensive Caring: Reminding Families They Matter. Harvey Max Chochinov. *Journal of Palliative Medicine*, 2024;27(2):152–155. Reprinted with permission from Mary Ann Liebert, Inc. publishers.

Abstract
Families often struggle with feelings of helplessness and futility in supporting suffering loved ones. Healthcare providers face similar struggles

when patients' ailments aren't readily fixable. Intensive Caring describes an approach to being with suffering, inspired by the words of Dame Cicely Saunders who said "you matter because you are you, and you matter to the last moment of your life." Intensive Caring describes how to affirm patients matter, comprised of non-abandonment, taking an interest in the patient as a person, knowing what is possible, guiding families towards viable opportunities, dignity affirming tone, and therapeutic humility. While originally conceived for healthcare providers, its applications for families supporting suffering loved ones remains to be explored.

* * * * *

An old family friend recently took me aside, lamenting how useless he felt visiting his wife in hospice, now facing progressive physical and cognitive decline. "All I do is just hold her hand and try to feed her a little. We often fall asleep in front of the television. It just doesn't feel like enough."

Introduction

Families of patients often encounter a sense of futility, feeling like helpless bystanders in the face of medical circumstances largely beyond their control.[1] Although health care professionals have the advantage of knowing various therapeutic measures and maneuvers to consider each step of the way, families are less fortunate in that regard. Although health care professionals can usually find something to do, families must often settle for "just showing up," witnessing suffering whose reach extends well beyond the grasp of their caring and protective embrace.

In many ways, this mirrors the experience of health care professionals who sometimes face suffering that cannot be fixed. In those instances, like families, they find themselves feeling hopeless and impotent; that despite their best efforts, "it just doesn't feel like enough."

Intensive Caring is a recently coined term, referring to a detailed approach outlining how health care professionals can address suffering that isn't fixable.[2] It takes its inspiration from the teachings of Dame Cicely Saunders, founder of the modern hospice movement and palliative care, who famously said, "you matter because you are you, and you matter to the last moment of your life."[3]

Intensive Caring describes how to show patients they matter and offers ways of being with them that displaces futility with empowerment, and counters therapeutic nihilism with empirically based approaches that are essential and effective for patients who feel unworthy of support, or that their ongoing existence is inconsequential. Although Intensive Caring was designed with health care providers in mind, how it applies to family caregivers, who feel their support for loved ones is not enough, bears examination.

Why Families Matter

According to the AARP report Caring in the US 2015, 43.5 million adults in the United States have provided unpaid care to an adult or a child in the last 13 months: in about 80% of instances, to an adult age 50 years or greater.[4] Sixty percent of these informal caregivers are female, with an average age of 49 years old. These caregivers spend an average of 24.4 hours a week providing care to their loved one. Nearly one-quarter provide 41 or more hours of care a week, with those caring for a spouse/partner providing an average of 44.6 hours a week.

The nature of tasks they engage in are varied, including food preparation, housekeeping, laundry, transportation, and giving medication; feeding, dressing, grooming, walking, bathing, and assistance toileting; getting in and out of beds and chairs, or using technology; coordinating physician visits or managing financial matters. Caregivers also report holding significant decision-making authority, including monitoring of the care recipient's condition, and adjusting care; communicating with health care professionals on behalf of the care recipient; acting as an advocate for the care recipient with care providers, community services, or government agencies.

The value of services provided by informal caregivers has steadily increased over the last decade, with an estimated economic value of $600 billion in 2021, up from $470 billion in 2017 and $450 billion in 2009.[5]

If ever there was doubt about the importance of families in health care, the coronavirus disease 2019 (COVID-19) pandemic settled that once and for all. With families barred from the bedside, the health care system buckled under an untenable strain. Physical tasks and emotional support normally shouldered by family members fell to health care providers or, tragically, fell to the wayside.[6-8] Millions died with about 81% of deaths occurring in those 65 years old or greater.[9] This abject suffering was compounded by assaults

Table 20.1. Elements of Intensive Caring (Adapted for Family Caregivers)[2]

- Nonabandonment
  - Committed, quality connection
  - Ongoing support
- Taking an interest in person for who they are
  - Enhance empathy, respect, connectedness
  - Affirm worth of who they are, were, or tried to be, and what they achieved or tried to accomplish
  - Reminding health care providers who their loved one is or was as a person
- Knowing What is Possible: Holding/containing hope
  - Finding hope for psychological, spiritual, and physical comfort
  - Hope for minimal suffering and a peaceful death
  - Finding meaning and purpose in
    - Relationships
    - Imparting words/sentiments that need to be shared, such as reconciliation, forgiveness, love, and affirmation of feelings
    - Sharing reminiscence
    - Dignity affirming tone/therapeutic presence
  - Being compassionate and empathic
  - Being respectful and nonjudgmental
  - Being genuine and authentic
  - Being trustworthy
  - Being fully present
  - Valuing intrinsic worth of the person
- Therapeutic humility
  - Tolerate ambiguity of the situation
  - Trust in the process
  - Avoid the need to fix.

---

on personhood, intense isolation, and fractured dignity, with families unable to provide support or offer affirmation to patients yearning to feel they still mattered.[10]

Elements of Intensive Caring

Like health care professionals, family members may feel they have little to offer in response to patient suffering that cannot be fixed (Table 20.1). A key tenet of Intensive Caring is **non-abandonment,** which demands committed, ongoing caring, even when patients no longer care about themselves. Dame Cicely wrote "suffering is only intolerable when nobody cares."[3] Thus, family members must appreciate their continued presence is vital in mitigating suffering and decreasing feelings of isolation. It affirms for their loved one they matter enough for them to be there, to show up, to accompany.

Connectedness has long been shown to be one the greatest protective measures in preventing suicide, in that it creates a sense of belonging and a feeling of being valued.[11] Hence, families must appreciate that nonabandonment, remaining involved and connected with their loved ones, is nothing less than life sustaining.

Another component of Intensive Caring **is taking a keen interest in who the patient is as a person.** For family members, this means sustaining a connection with loved ones based on who they are, and not—as typifies health care professionals—focused on their ailment. Family members are ideally positioned to do this, given they know the patient's life story, interests, values, beliefs, accomplishments, challenges, and fears; in other words, their connection, shared history, and affiliation predate illness and all its various incumbrances. Familial ties are usually based on appreciation for who someone is, rather than simply the functions they fulfill.

It is that essence or what illness cannot break—often the very foundation of the relationship itself—that families recognize, value, and affirm, thus reinforcing the patient's worth as someone who still matters.[12] In so doing, they enable patients to connect with the core of who they are, who they were, or who they are striving to be, staving off feelings of despair or thoughts of early death. This means that families relate in ways that simply cannot be replicated, further attesting to the profound, supportive role they play.[13]

Besides helping patients feel connected with, and appreciated for, who they are, families play a vital advocacy role, which includes reminding health care providers who their patient is or was as a person. This is a profound responsibility, which families are uniquely positioned to fulfill. By doing so, they ensure the patient is seen as more than the embodiment of their ailment, but appreciated as a unique, individual human being.

Our studies of the Patient Dignity Question (PDQ), which asks "what do I need to know about you as a person to give you the best care possible," have demonstrated that when patients are seen through the lens of personhood, health care providers are able to feel greater empathy, connectedness, and respect, and gain an appreciation for the patient's values and goals of care.[14] By reminding health care providers who their patient is as a person, families ensure that their loved ones are truly seen, hence safeguarding and preserving their innate dignity.

Another element of Intensive Caring is **knowing what is possible and holding or containing hope.** For patients nearing end of life, hope often resides in the domain of meaning and purpose.[15,16] Family members who question their utility—that what they do "just doesn't feel like enough"—likely do not appreciate their role in facilitating meaning and purpose. This can include helping loved ones find meaning in pursuit of psychological, spiritual, and physical comfort, and for those near the end of life, a peaceful death. Meaning and purpose can be nurtured through connections with people or things that matter. This may include affirming all that needs saying has been said or bears repeating.

Clinical approaches that enable this kind of information sharing have been shown to mitigate psychological distress, enhance end-of-life experience, while empowering families.[14,17,18] Reminiscence can affirm the importance of patients' stories, helping them integrate those experiences into the entirety of their lives.[19] Towards the end of life, there may be a shared sense of meaning and purpose as families and patients prepare one another for separation imposed by death.

My mother's final year of life was not easy, and fraught with challenges associated with multiple comorbidities as she approached her final days. That year was marked, however, by countless games of cards, cups of tea, and conversations; and stories of her past, many visitors, and expressions of appreciation and love. Although this was excruciatingly difficult at times, it was not without meaning or purpose, which was to help her live as best she could until she died, and to prepare our family for life without her.

Intensive Caring requires a tone of care that is dignity affirming. We have studied this tone among health care providers, which we labeled **Therapeutic Presence.**[20] The latter consists of being compassionate and empathic, being respectful and nonjudgmental, being genuine and authentic, being trustworthy, being fully present, and valuing the intrinsic worth of the patient. From the family's perspective, this tone can be conveyed by virtue of love, caring, and concern; in other words, mere presence, independent of what is said or done, can impart Intensive Caring.

Hence, families need not feel uncomfortable not knowing what to say, mindful that tone of care speaks volumes without uttering a single word. Recalling my family friend: holding hands, being concerned, and being present conveyed a poignant and vital message; that the decades long connection between them was unbreakable and would endure. This tone of caring affirms patients' worth, provides respect, while confirming they still matter.

Within the realm of human suffering, some problems simply defy repair. This can engender feelings of helplessness and an inclination to withdraw.

When cure or the elimination of suffering is out of reach, feelings of failure and falling short—that what is being done does not feel like enough—are bound to emerge. This is why Intensive Caring includes **therapeutic humility**, which requires an ability to relinquish the need to fix, along with being able to tolerate ambiguity, accepting and honoring the patient as expert, and trusting in the process.[20]

The implications of therapeutic humility for families are profound. It insists families yield the notion of fixing, appreciating that while eliminating suffering is not always possible, providing comfort is. Intensive Caring offers families a way of being with patients, shaping an optimal response to their loved one's anguish. Therapeutic humility accepts the uncertainties of this process, trusting that presence and affirmation provide a space to bear witness, to validate, and offer the surest path toward healing.

As illness claimed more and more of those features she affiliated with sense of self and core identity, my mother's suffering began to mount. Not being able to entertain, not being able to cook, lacking the energy to engage in pleasurable activities sapped her of vitality and a sense of being the person she once was. Although our family understood the inevitability of her death, we remained ever present, ever engaged, reminding her that she was and would always remain cherished in our hearts. Although the anguish of departing from those she loved was impenetrable, she was calmest and most herself when able to hold us close within her watchful gaze.

Conclusions

Connections between family members vary, as does the capacity to lean in and support ill loved ones. Willingness to do so is usually shaped by personal predisposition and resources, historical complexities, and current relationship dynamics. Even those inclined may feel overwhelmed by feelings of helplessness and a sense of futility. That is why tenets of Intensive Caring must inform how we conceive the role of family caregivers. Doing so will accomplish the following:

1. It will help family caregivers embrace their role, helping them understand the profound influence continued presence has in the well-being of their loved one.

2. It will lessen family member suffering by helping them maintain their core identity within the relationship, which is to protect, comfort, and accompany those they care about.

3. It will improve family caregiver emotional health, given helplessness and hopelessness are frequent harbingers of more severe mental disturbances such as depression and anxiety.[21]

4. It will improve patient outcomes, given they are the beneficiaries of family caregivers' physical, emotional, and spiritual support and advocacy.

5. It will support the efforts of individual health care providers and health care systems, given neither can replace nor replicate the role family caregivers offer patients confronting illness.

Just as it applies to health care professionals, Intensive Caring, the therapeutic derivative of Dame Cicely's "You matter because you are you," provides families a way of being with loved ones who are suffering. As with health care providers, Intensive Caring empowers family caregivers to target achievable goals, focused on myriad ways of affirming that their loved one matters.[22] It has been over 50 years since Dame Cicely shared the wisdom underpinning this approach. Families can invoke Intensive Caring, in the service of caring for loved ones, knowing that what they are doing matters, and that their continued presence, involvement, and support are, absolutely and undeniably, enough.

References

1. Kristjanson LJ, Aoun S. Palliative care for families: remembering the hidden patients. *Can J Psychiatry.* 2004;49:359–365.
2. Chochinov HM. Intensive caring: reminding patients they matter. *J Clin Oncol.* 2023;41:2884–2887.
3. Cicely Saunders quotes. https://www.azquotes.com/author/20332-Cicely_Saunders.
4. Caregiving in the US. Research Report June 2015 NAC and AARP Public Policy Institute. https://www.aarp.org/content/dam/aarp/ppi/2015/caregiving-in-the-united-states-2015-executive-summary-revised.pdf (last accessed July 28, 2023).
5. Caregiver Statistics: Demographics. Family Caregiver Alliance. https://www.caregiver.org/resource/caregiver-statistics-demographics/ (last accessed July 28, 2023).
6. Hugelius K, Harada N, Marutani M. Consequences of visiting restrictions during the COVID-19 pandemic: an integrative review. *Int J Nurs Stud.* 2021;121:104000.
7. Gergerich E, Mallonee J, Gherardi S, et al. Strengths and struggles for families involved in hospice care during the COVID-19 pandemic. *J Soc Work End of Life Palliat Care.* 2021;17:198–217.

8. Silvera GA, Wolf JA, Stanowski A, Studer Q. The influence of COVID-19 visitation restrictions on patient experience and safety outcomes: a critical role for subjective advocates. *Patient Exp J.* 2021;8:30–39.
9. Deaths by Select Demographic and Geographic Characteristics. Centers for Disease Control and Prevention. https://www.cdc.gov/nchs/nvss/vsrr/covid_weekly/index.htm (last accessed July 28, 2023).
10. Chochinov HM, Bolton J, Sareen J. Death, dying, and dignity in the time of the COVID-19 pandemic. *J Palliat Med.* 2020;23:1294–1295.
11. Zareian B, Klonsky ED. Connectedness and suicide. In: Page AC, Stritzke WGK, eds. *Alternatives to Suicide.* Academic Press; 2020:135–158.
12. Chochinov HM. Michael J. Fox gives patients hope there may be a place that illness doesn't touch. Globe and Mail. https://www.theglobeandmail.com/opinion/article-michael-j-fox-gives-patients-hope-there-may-be-a-place-that-illness/ (last accessed July 28, 2023).
13. Keeley MP. Family communication at the end of life. *Behav Sci.* 2017;7:45.
14. Chochinov HM, McClement S, Hack T, et al. Eliciting personhood within clinical practice: effects on patients, families, and health care providers. *J Pain Symptom Manage.* 2015;4:974–980.
15. Chochinov HM, Wilson KG, Enns M, Lander S. Depression, hopelessness, and suicidal ideation in the terminally ill. *Psychosomatics.* 1998;39:366–370.
16. Breitbart W, Rosenfeld B, Pessin H, et al. Depression, hopelessness, and desire for hastened death in terminally ill patients with cancer. *JAMA.* 2000;284:2907–2911.
17. Chochinov HM. *Dignity Therapy: Final Words for Final Days.* Oxford University Press; 2011.
18. McClement S, Chochinov HM, Hack T, et al. Dignity therapy: family member perspectives. *J Palliat Med.* 2007;10:1076–1082.
19. Westerhof GJ, Bohlmeijer ET. Celebrating fifty years of research and applications in reminiscence and life review: state of the art and new directions. *J Aging Stud.* 2014;29:107–114.
20. Chochinov HM, McClement SE, Hack TF, et al. Health care provider communication: an empirical model of therapeutic effectiveness. *Cancer.* 2013;119:1706–1713.
21. Kendler KS, Hettema JM, Butera F, et al. Life event dimensions of loss, humiliation, entrapment, and danger in the prediction of onsets of major depression and generalized anxiety. *Arch Gen Psychiatry.* 2003;60:789–796.
22. Chochinov HM. *Dignity in Care: The Human Side of Medicine.* Oxford University Press; 2022.

21

Fractured Personhood, Suicide, and Lessons from Those Nearing Death

I'm not sure exactly when it happened, but somewhere along the way of doing palliative care research came the realization that our studies and the things we are trying to understand, resonate across all of medicine. While palliative care offers an intriguing vantage point for examining what happens to people in the face of adversity, the insights gleaned from these studies apply not only to end of life, but to all of life.

This article on fractured personhood is a good example. While I first landed on this idea relative to palliative care, the connection between a state of brokenness and suicidal ideation lends itself to broader examination. I am now launching a study inviting patients who have contemplated or attempted suicide to reflect on fractured personhood, and the extent to which the notion of brokenness factors into their wish to die. Other innovations and insights have moved beyond palliative care, with Dignity Therapy, for example, now being applied to patients with earlier-stage cancers, dementia, and serious mental illness. The Patient Dignity Inventory, while originating in palliative care, is now a gold standard for tracking dignity and dignity-related distress in various areas of medicine (including psychiatry, acute care, geriatric medicine, and intensive care).

Understanding the potential reach of this work has changed my knowledge translation goals and priorities. While I've given over 550 talks during my career, most have been for palliative care or cancer care professional audiences. In my third act I hope to reach a more general audience representing a broader scope of medicine. My most recent book, Dignity in Care: The Human Side of Medicine, *was written with that intent, targeting anyone having patient contact. This year, the Faculty of Medicine gifted a copy of that book to all the incoming medical students (see* Chapter 37). *My inscription in each book encouraged them to be more than human-body*

In Search of Dignity. Harvey Max Chochinov, Oxford University Press. © Oxford University Press 2025.
DOI: 10.1093/9780197805145.003.0021

mechanics, and to strive to be healers. Helpful advice, I hope, for young people just starting their training in medicine.

Fractured Personhood, Suicide, and Lessons from Those Nearing Death. Harvey Max Chochinov. *Journal of Palliative Medicine*, 2023;26(8):1037–1039. Reprinted with permission from Mary Ann Liebert, Inc. publishers.

Abstract
Sometimes dying patients teach us things that apply across the entirety of the life cycle. There is a significant literature indicating that some patients toward end of life covet an earlier, or hastened, death. Many of the things that move patients toward a wish to die can be subsumed under the rubric of *fractured personhood*. This idea describes a state of *brokenness*, causing people to feel they are no longer the person they once were, and that the person they have become is no longer worthy of living. This article explores the idea of fractured personhood, and how this concept might inform our understanding of self-harm and suicide within the general population.

Introduction

Conducting research in palliative care has taught me that dying patients often reveal insights that apply across the entirety of human experience.[1] For those nearing death, meaning, purpose, feeling affirmed for who they are, and connections with others are paramount.[2] Dying, however, does not have a monopoly on those issues, which are vital throughout life although perhaps more pressing or amplified as time is running out. This leads one to speculate whether the dynamic moving terminally ill patients toward a wish to die might provide insights regarding suicide and self-harm across the entire life cycle.

Our studies of the terminally ill demonstrate strong associations between depression, hopelessness, and a desire for death.[3] Similarly associations between depression, hopelessness, and suicide throughout life are well documented.[4] A deeper dive into the psychological, existential, and spiritual antecedents of a wish to die reveals dying patients disclose struggles that cut to the core of who they are as persons. For those coveting hastened death, the inability to carry out meaningful activities, loss of autonomy, diminished agency, and loss of dignity figure prominently.[5]

Each describe influences that can cause people to feel they are no longer the person they once were. In other words, wanting to die emerges within a state of fractured personhood, marked by dissatisfaction, contempt, and rejection of who they are, relative to who they were or want to be, ultimately making life intolerable.

Looking Toward Suicide

How might those insights regarding the fragility of personhood apply to self-harm and suicide beyond the confines of terminal illness? While facing death is the quintessential existential trauma, trauma in all its various forms heightens the risk of suicide. Sexual and other interpersonal traumas (such as rape, sexual assault, intimate partner violence, spousal abuse, and child abuse) are all significantly associated with suicide attempts in both men and women, even when controlling for sociodemographic characteristics and mental disorders.[6] There is also strong evidence that the number of traumatic events experienced is positively associated with increased risk of suicide attempts, indicating a dose–response effect of exposure to trauma.

Even witnessing traumatic events, such as bad injury, rape, physical attack, and physical abuse, appears to heighten the risk of suicide.[7] Like at end of life, perhaps patients exposed to trauma experience an assault on integrity of personhood, causing them to feel they are no longer the person they once were or the person they want to be. Trauma, whether interpersonal or non-interpersonal, threatens agency, seeing us confront forces beyond our control, capable of overwhelming our most intense, although futile, resistance. Despite any prior sense of unassailable autonomy or self-reliance—pleasant, although fleeting, illusions of youth—trauma thrusts us into a new reality that shatters those precepts.

Those experiencing sexual assault discover that they can be overpowered, leaving them feeling fragile and weak; those experiencing intimate partner violence or child abuse discover that familial connections do not necessarily avert violence, leaving them feeling defenseless; the incarcerated learn that they cannot will their freedom, leaving them feeling trapped; the bereft discover that love cannot protect those they cherish from the ravages of illness or calamity, leaving them feeling helpless; and those bearing witness to trauma learn that their abhorrence and horror carry no sway whatsoever, leaving them feeling like impotent bystanders.

Feeling fragile, weak, defenseless, trapped, helpless, and impotent are at complete odds with the person they once were or the person they want to be. And so, in directing their rage inward, they feel compelled to destroy the person they can no longer tolerate—that person being themselves.[8]

The great American suicidologist Edwin Shneidman wrote that the frustration or blocking of certain human needs accounts for a large percentage of suicides.[9] The intensity of needs, he posited, determines the degree of perturbation leading to lethality. Among others, those needs implicate ruptured relationships, fractured control, and assault of self-image—all consistent with a state of fractured personhood—leaving patients feeling less intact and no longer the person they once were.

Aging can threaten integrity of personhood, requiring accommodation to waning autonomy, vitality, and agency, with the inability to adapt likely accounting for a heightened risk of suicide.[10] For those suddenly thrust into a state of fractured personhood, by way of illness, calamity, or trauma, feeling intact, autonomous, and resilient sometimes yields to brokenness, marked by a sense of inadequacy, fragility, self-loathing, and a compulsion to self-destruct.

The interpersonal-psychological theory of suicidal behavior proposes that an individual will not die by suicide unless there is both the desire and the ability to do so.[11] This theory holds that desire to die is driven by perceived burdensomeness and a sense of not belonging or social alienation.

For dying patients, this feeling of being a burden correlates highly with a desire for hastened death.[12] Patients may feel a shadow of their former selves, and that their lives no longer matter.[13] Toward end of life, coveting death aligns with perceived lack of social support[3] and emotional decathexis from those previously held dear.

Regarding suicide in general, low belongingness and social alienation often merge with self-deprecation, wherein patients see themselves lacking value, having nothing worthwhile to contribute. Thus, feeling unworthy of connection or belonging are painful elements of brokenness, aligning with a state of fractured personhood.

Conclusion

The notion of fractured personhood, gleaned from patients nearing death, offers a way of formulating, and perhaps preventing, mitigating, and

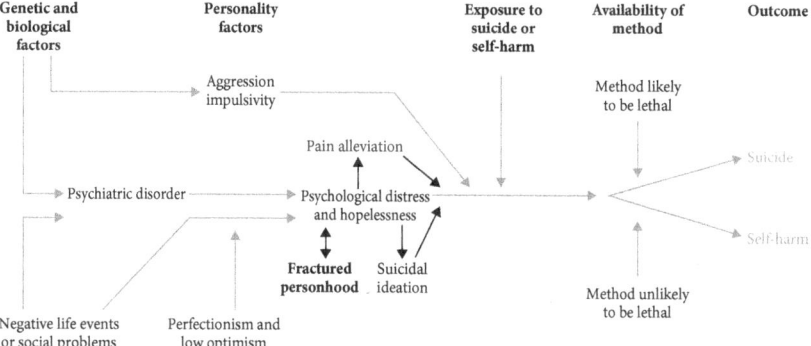

Figure 21.1 Key risk factors for self-harm and suicide.[14] Adapted from Keith Hawton, Kate E.A. Saunders, Rory C. O'Connor. Self-harm and suicide in adolescents. Lancet 2012;379:2373–2382.

addressing suicidality across the life cycle (Figure 21.1).[14] In palliative care, suffering, brokenness, and fractured personhood are ideally addressed by Intensive Caring, comprised of core elements including non-abandonment, affirmation, and reframing vulnerability, dependency, and fragility as part of our collective humanity.[13]

Fractured personhood needs to be explored as a means of unravelling the psychological, existential, and spiritual complexities underpinning self-harm, suicide, and the wish to die. Although these insights are arrived at from studying dying patients, they may nevertheless inform our way of understanding those for whom death represents a tragic, often violent, premature, and self-imposed departure.

References

1. Chochinov HM, Breitbart WS, eds. *The Handbook of Psychiatry in Palliative Medicine: Psychosocial Care for the Terminally Ill.* 3rd ed. Oxford University Press; 2022.
2. Byock I. *Dying Well: Peace and Possibilities at the End of Life.* Riverhead Books; 1997.
3. Chochinov HM, Wilson K, Enns M, et al. Desire for death in the terminally ill. *Am J Psychiatry.* 1995;152:1185–1191.
4. Ribeiro J, Huang X, Fox K, et al. Depression and hopelessness as risk factors for suicide ideation, attempts and death: meta-analysis of longitudinal studies. *Br J Psychiatry.* 2018;212:279–286.
5. Chochinov HM, Hack T, Hassard T, et al. The landscape of distress in the terminally ill. *J Pain Sympt Manag.* 2009;38:641–649.
6. Belik SL, Stein MB, Asmundson GJ, et al. Relation between traumatic events and suicide attempts in Canadian military personnel. *Can J Psychiatry.* 2009;54:93–104.
7. Belik SL, Cox BJ, Stein MB, et al. Traumatic events and suicidal behavior results from a National Mental Health Survey. *J Nervous Mental Dis.* 2007;195:342–349.

8. Chochinov HM. Depression is a liar. *Globe and Mail.* https://www.theglobeandmail.com/opinion/article-depression-is-a-liar/ (published May 3, 2023; last accessed May 8, 2023).

9. *Psychological Factors in Suicide.* ncbi.nlm.nih.gov/books/NBK223745/ (last accessed February 10, 2023).

10. Conejero I, Olié E, Courtet P, et al. Suicide in older adults: current perspectives. *Clin Interv Aging.* 2018;13:691–699.

11. Ribeiro JD, Joiner TE. The interpersonal-psychological theory of suicidal behavior: current status and future directions. *J Clin Psychol.* 2009;65:1291–1299.

12. *Third Annual Report on Medical Assistance in Dying in Canada 2021.* Health Canada; 2022.

13. Chochinov HM. Intensive caring: reminding patients they matter. *J Clin Oncol.* 2023;41(16):2884–2887. doi:10.1200/JCO.23.00042

14. Hawton K, Saunders KEA, O'Connor TC. Self-harm and suicide in adolescents. *Lancet.* 2012;379:2373–2382.

22

The Secret Is Out

Patients Are People with Feelings That Matter

When he was 8 years old, Francis Peabody and his younger brother John were taken on vacation to Florence, Italy. While there, both boys were stricken with typhoid; while Francis survived, his brother did not. It is believed the death of his brother played a role in Francis's decision to choose medicine as a career. He went on to become a celebrated teacher at Harvard Medical School and made significant contributions to the study of poliomyelitis and, ironically, typhoid. He rose rapidly in the academic ranks, was appointed Professor of Medicine at Harvard, and the following year was named Director of the Thorndike Memorial Laboratory and Physician-in-Chief of the Fourth Medical Service at Boston City Hospital. His iconic career ended prematurely when he died 6 years later at the age of 45 of metastatic stomach cancer.

Had he lived a few years more, he may have shared the Nobel Prize with his friend George R. Minot for the discovery of liver therapy for pernicious anemia. Despite those illustrious contributions, what Francis Weld Peabody is best remembered for nearly 100 years after his death is being the man who wrote what is considered one of the best and most widely quoted articles on patient care ever published. "The Care of the Patient" appeared in JAMA in 1927. In it, he says, "The good physician knows his patients through and through, and his knowledge is bought dearly. Time, sympathy and understanding must be lavishly dispensed, but the reward is to be found in that personal bond which forms the greatest satisfaction of the practice of medicine." And he concludes with these words, which have become iconic in medicine: "One of the essential qualities of the clinician is interest in humanity, for the secret of the care of the patient is in caring for the patient."

The title of my article in this chapter takes its inspiration from Dr. Peabody's famous essay. The longevity of his message speaks to the power of well-crafted words, words that capture essential wisdom and

In Search of Dignity. Harvey Max Chochinov, Oxford University Press. © Oxford University Press 2025.
DOI: 10.1093/9780197805145.003.0022

retain their strength despite the passage of time. Words matter. When we get them right, they can leave an indelible mark that shapes our thinking and changes the way we see and respond to the world. So, invoking the spirit of Dr. Francis Peabody, I remind everyone working in medicine that "The Secret Is Out: Patients Are People with Feelings That Matter."

The Secret Is Out: Patients Are People with Feelings That Matter. Harvey Max Chochinov. *Palliative & Supportive Care*, 2013;11(4):287–288. Reproduced with permission of Cambridge University Press.

In his famous address to Harvard medical students in the fall of 1925, Dr. Frances Peabody stated: "the secret of the care of the patient is in caring for the patient." While few would argue the wisdom of this beautifully crafted, and often quoted aphorism, medicine struggles to uphold this simple credo. It would seem straightforward enough, and yet repeatedly, and for the most part, unwittingly, we still sometimes manage to get it wrong. Too often, patients bemoan feeling processed, not really being heard; suddenly being defined according to what they have as a patient and not who they are as a person.

I was recently discussing this with one of my colleagues, a physician who has been in practice for nearly 30 years and holds several cross appointments within the faculty of medicine. While our discussion began on a rather cerebral note—the culture of contemporary health care, the role of technology, mounting workloads and crushing time pressures—things turned personal when she began to reflect on her own experiences as a patient. Of note, even the subtleties of patienthood, she said, could be abrasive; being examined, talking with certain doctors, "and the gowns . . . the gowns are a problem." And yet, through the lens of patienthood, these things are completely routine, even mundane. But through a personhood lens, they look entirely different.

Take the medical gown for instance. The moment someone enters a hospital, their usual attire and rationale for choosing it—comfort, allure, status, affiliation—is replaced by a drab gown, theoretically meant to fasten at the back, Designed for EAse of Defecation (D.E.A.D.) being an appropriate acronym, given that people, under normal circumstances, would not want to be caught dead wearing them.

And yet, the instant one is hospitalized, the overarching schema, world-wide, regarding clothing is organized around bodily waste. For *persons*, clothing is about pride, modesty, an expression of our unique individuality; values that are critical in maintaining our sense of self and personhood. Entering hospital begins an insidious transformation from person to patient, wherein those values are suddenly displaced. Individuality must yield to uniformity, and modesty, for anyone who has ever worn such a gown knows all too well, is left behind.

Being cloaked in a gown that is incapable of hiding one's nakedness has existential consequences. So too does having to relinquish control over who sees, probes, and evaluates the integrity, or lack thereof, of one's body. While nakedness describes a state of not being clothed, it also conveys the notion of lacking protection and hence being vulnerable.

> *Had I but served my God with half the zeal*
> *I served my King, he would not in mine age*
> *Have left me naked to mine enemies.*
> (*Cardinal Wolsey, Henry VIII*)

Reflecting on a recent visit to her medical oncologist, a woman with metastatic breast cancer reported feeling upset with the medical student who examined her mastectomy scar. Without intending her to feel "naked to mine enemies," the assault she felt was nevertheless real. Perhaps it was his first opportunity to see what a chest wall looks like following the removal of a cancerous breast tumor, or to carefully palpate the remnants of a suture line. But the patient's response leaves no doubt that the scar being examined extended much deeper than any physical injury. While the student was likely mindful of anatomical landmarks and signs of infection or abnormal healing, what may not have been on his radar was the experiential landscape of living with Stage IV, terminal breast cancer; a landscape invariably marked by fear, sadness and loss.

Without being attentive to the emotional consequences of illness and disease, even technically competent care runs the risk of inflicting similar harm. This accounts for why patients sometimes find health care encounters abrasive; or why, accurate diagnostic and therapeutic steps notwithstanding, medicine can fall short of meeting patients' needs.

> *It is the disease of not listening,*
> *the malady of not marking,*
> *that I am troubled withal.*
>
> *(Falstaff, Henry IV, Part 2)*

Optimal therapeutic effectiveness—perhaps a modern-day version of the secret of caring for the patient—requires that health care professionals provide the right care, consisting of appropriate evidence-based approaches, within a context that feels safe for patients and families.[1] But it also demands, by way of invoking aspects of our own humanity—such as compassion, empathy, respect, and humility—that we pay attention to *persons.*

One can only speculate on how Peabody might have responded to this contemporary rejigging of his conventional wisdom. While it remains focused on caring, it speaks to the centrality of persons and the notion of personhood within this therapeutic calculus. After all, patients are people; and people have feelings; and those feelings matter. Admittedly, nowhere near as eloquent as Peabody, but hopefully of some utility. Patients are people with feelings that matter.[a] And now the secret is out.

Reference

1. Chochinov HM, McClement SE, Hack TF, et al. Health care provider communication: an empirical model of therapeutic effectiveness. *Cancer.* 2013;119:1703–1713.

---

[a] In case there are any medical students reading this, it is worth committing to memory. Yes, it is core.

23

Death, Time, and the Theory of Relativity

I enjoy learning. About 7 years after completing my psychiatry residency, I began my doctoral studies in the Faculty of Community Health Sciences at the University of Manitoba. At the time I was a grantee of Project on Death in America (PDIA), and this educational opportunity struck me as a perfect professional development strategy, which was one of the expectations of being a PDIA Soros Faculty Scholar.

Being a student can be anxiety provoking, especially when it involves vocational training with so much of one's future and security hanging in the balance. But being a mature student is entirely different. There is something luxurious and even self-indulgent when learning is entirely about personal challenge and intellectual growth, absent those unsettling feelings of risk or uncertainty. Intellectual nourishment included learning about public policy, qualitative and quantitative methodology, epidemiology, and biostatistics. While I've always been drawn to literature and the arts, I also appreciate the intricacies of number crunching and its exquisite logic.

A concept I struggled with, however, was quality-adjusted life years (QALYs). My difficulty was not mathematical, but philosophical. The QALY is a generic measure of disease burden, which considers the quality and the quantity of life lived. One QALY is the equivalent of 1 year in perfect health. Hence, less quality equates to less valuable time lived (e.g., living 1 year with a 50% disability yields a 6-month valuation). In certain instances, QALYs have been used to inform treatment decisions, resource allocation, program evaluation, and priority setting. The problem, however, is the assumption that less ability means less value. For anyone living with a disability, the implications are stark: From an actuarial perspective and considering the bottom line, your life isn't worth as much.

Applying this concept to palliative care is equally fraught. As people approach death, quality of life declines. Applying a QALY rationale means that as quality ebbs, life—from an empirical, Orwellian perspective—becomes worthless and dispensable. Those of us well acquainted with death and dying know that as health deteriorates, perception of time becomes distorted

In Search of Dignity. Harvey Max Chochinov, Oxford University Press. © Oxford University Press 2025.
DOI: 10.1093/9780197805145.003.0023

and the valuation of time becomes distended. Toward the end, time begins to shrug off its cosmic moorings. The subtleties and nuances of that time interval are hard to describe and yet—for anyone who has experienced the death of a loved one—hard to forget. Conversations may feel more intense or urgent, interactions more poignant; memories become indelibly etched. Patients facing death recall loved ones who died decades earlier, with the quality of that death shaping their expectations of how their own dying will unfold.

Those who have sat vigil at the bedside of a dying loved one know the precious quality of time, and the intense savoring of whatever time is left. As my sister Ellen was in her final days, our family spelled each other off, ensuring she was never alone and that her final breath would be in the presence of those who loved her. Given my parents' fatigue, my sister Brenda and I decided we would stay the night together in her hospital room. I'll carry that memory forever. It was the first time in decades and would be the last time all three children would sleep under one roof. It meant something to all of us; something one can't put a price on.

Death, Time, and the Theory of Relativity. Harvey Max Chochinov. *Journal of Pain and Symptom Management*, 2011;42(3):460–463. Reprinted with permission from Elsevier.

Abstract
Many people believe that spending large amounts of money on end-of-life care is unjustified and even irrational. This fails to recognize that the value of time, particularly quality time, appears to increase as death draws near. Paying for treatment that merely allows patients and families to avoid confronting the inevitability of death is wrong. However, palliative care, which can bolster the quality of a patient's remaining days, provides benefits that extend to the family and beyond. How can the notion of time gaining value toward the end of life be incorporated into conventional cost-benefit analyses? A standard QALY (Quality Adjusted Life Years) is the product of quality of life and time, without adjusting for any change in the value of time. An additional variable—a Valuation Index (Palliative) (or VIP)—needs to be factored into the equation, providing a rational explanation for what otherwise might be deemed irrational spending. When one recognizes the

multitude of important things that happen as people approach the very end of life, the numbers start to add up.

Time Is Relative

According to Einstein's celebrated theorem, time is relative. To prove his point, Einstein performed an ingenious thought experiment, involving a stationary observer, a passing train with an outer transparent wall, and a passenger tossing a ball in the direction of the moving train. While the ingredients of this experiment are innocent enough, their combination stymied Newtonian laws of motion, unhinging time itself from its stalwart cosmic moorings. As implausible as it seems, Einstein discovered that time expands or contracts relative to speed; while a person situated on earth will experience several days, a person traveling in a very fast spaceship experiences mere minutes or hours. In theory, if someone could travel at the speed of light, time would come to a standstill, leaving them trapped in timelessness.

While based on different theoretical considerations, people who work closely with the dying and anyone who has ever watched someone they love die, know that time is relative. People caught in the gravity of approaching death encounter a profound distortion of how time is experienced and valued. Each moment becomes increasingly precious as death draws near; while for the rest of the world, the clock marks time at its usual pace, with its usual indifference.

Consider the following thought experiment. Imagine yourself—or recall being—at the bedside of a dying loved one. What value would you place on being able to extend this time—with some assurances around lack of pain and suffering—by a month, perhaps just a week or even as little as a day? I assume it is difficult to arrive at an answer stated in terms of absolutes, given that the offer and what is at stake seem beyond measure, if not priceless. The results of this thought experiment suggest that time, and the value of quality time, changes in proximity to death.

There is evidence to support this notion of heightened value of time toward the end of life.[1] Various studies, using time tradeoff or standard gamble techniques, have shown that patients who are ill tend to overvalue their current health, relative to those who are well.[2] Furthermore, as death draws near, demand for more medical care and a willingness to pay for it appear to increase, even when the return on this investment—in terms of life extension—is marginal.[3] This increasing valuation of time has been posited as a partial explanation for rising medical care expenditures at the end of life.[4] Currently, about twenty percent of all health care costs are spent in the last six months of life.[5] If absolute worth can be inferred based on the price paid, it would appear that the relative value of time increases as time itself is running out.

Why Spend on the Dying?

There is much ambivalence about spending a lot of money on people who are dying. Health care economists suggest that, based on conventional cost-benefit considerations, the magnitude of this spending hardly seems prudent.[6] Few would argue that spending exorbitant amounts of money on treatments that essentially allow patients, families and health care providers to avoid confronting the inevitability of death is simply wrong. Such avoidance can also be costly. Patient-physician discussions about end-of-life wishes lower rates of intensive interventions (such as mechanical ventilation, resuscitation, or admissions to an intensive care unit), achieving better quality of life and reducing costs in the final weeks of life by as much as 35%.[7]

Spending on palliative care buys dying patients and their families a higher quality of life for whatever time they have remaining. While time is normally valued for what it allows the patient to do, "in palliative care, perhaps it is valued simply for what it allows the patient to 'be' . . ."[1(p 52)] And what the patient can "be" might very well begin to explain the heightened value of time toward death. Until the patient has died, he or she remains part of a human drama, whose ending has not quite yet been written. Time offers the possibility for final words, a last embrace, finding spiritual peace and, occasionally, even reconciliation.

We also know that "dying right" can mitigate protracted grief, and quell doubt, guilt and regret that linger in the wake of poor end-of-life care. While not often considered in cost-benefit analyses, aggressive non-palliative medical care is associated with worse patient quality of life and higher risk of major depressive disorder in bereaved caregivers. Longer hospice stays, on the other hand, are associated with better patient quality of life and better caregiver quality of life.[8]

There may be broader societal benefits, underscoring the value of end-of-life spending. Looking after the dying provides powerful assurance that care will be available for those whose turn to die has yet to come.[3] Such perpetual assurance could be framed in terms of end-of-life care costs being amortized over the course of a lifetime. How we treat our dying also defines who we are as a society. Insufficient spending would mean accepting that bad things are allowed to happen to people when they are most vulnerable. This would have a chilling effect on our collective quality of life, challenging the assumption that we live in a moral and just society.

Finally, given that no one would suggest the dying ought not to be looked after, it is worth comparing the costs of good palliative care, rather than less optimal alternatives. On this front, the numbers speak for themselves. Palliative care programs can reduce hospital and intensive care unit expenditures by clarifying the goals of care and assisting patients and families to select treatments that are consistent with those goals. Hospital-based palliative care consultation teams have also been shown to improve care for adults with serious illness, and do so with significant hospital cost savings.[9]

Crunching the Numbers

When all is said and done, considerable sums of money are spent on end-of-life care. Such spending is unwise if inconsistent with the goals of palliative care, whose raison d'etre is to improve quality of life for patients and families facing life-limiting illness. According to the World Health Organization, this can be achieved by early identification and impeccable assessment and treatment of pain and other problems, physical, psychosocial and spiritual.[10] Hence, spending that helps achieve these goals is justifiable, whether it be for neuroablative procedures to alleviate pain; radiation or chemotherapy to decrease tumor bulk causing symptom distress; or a period of ventilator support to enable final farewells.

Those who deem spending at the end-of-life irrational would argue that the amount and quality of time will always be confined within limits set by the underlying disease. Applying a standard Quality Adjusted Life Year (QALY) analysis, limited quality and limited time will always lead to pronouncements of "money poorly spent." But this analysis fails to recognize that the value of time is not fixed, and that even a limited amount of quality time can provide the patient, family and society a multitude of benefits, as described.

So how might we redress the QALY approach, to demonstrate rationality for this seemingly irrational spending? What is missing is the ability to ascribe higher value, for the reasons outlined, to time, recognizing that its value increases in proximity to death. This suggests the need for a valuation index, or VI (Palliative) or simply, VIP. If we assume that the ever-increasing value of time as one moves toward death follows a pattern of exponential growth (other growth models are possible), then VIP could be expressed as follows:

$$VIP = D^{t/m}$$

where t = ([prognosis at diagnosis] – [proximity to death]), and m is the length of time it would take to enhance valuation by a factor of D. For example, let us consider a gentleman with a prognosis of 24 months at the time of his diagnosis. If value doubled in seven months, as he steadily moves toward death, three months into the course of his illness, VIP would be:

$$VIP = 2^{(24-21)/7} = 2^{(3/7)} = 1:346$$

meaning that the third month into illness could theoretically be ascribed 34.6% more value than the corresponding month three months earlier (this, of course, is strictly meant as an illustration, given there is no empirical data to support what the exponential growth in value might be).

With a way of defining VIP, the adjustment to the QALY approach would look as follows:

$$\text{Palliative Adjusted Life Yardstick} (\text{PalY})$$
$$= QALY \times VIP$$
$$= QALY \times D^{t/m}$$
$$= V \times QI \times D^{t/m}$$

where QI is a quality index that ranges from 0 (death) to 1 (perfect state of health) and V is the value of one unit of healthy life (with time increments expressed in terms of years, months, weeks or days). (The term PalY [Palliative Care Yardstick], while not previously mathematically defined, was first introduced into the literature by Charles Normand.[6]) So for example, imagine that the gentleman previously described is now 13 months into his

illness, with a QI of 50% (half his baseline quality of life). The PalY calculation would look as follows:

$$PalY = V \times 0.5 \times 2^{(24-13)/7}$$
$$= V \times 0.5 \times 3.623$$
$$= 1:812\,V$$

whereas the QALY calculation would be:

$$QALY = V \times QI$$
$$= 0.5V$$

Notice that while a conventional QALY approach leads to a 50% reduction in
value, the PalY method indicates a total value of nearly double its original (in
spite of less-than-optimal quality of life), thereby providing rationale for significant end-of-life care expenditure—be it the cost of analgesics or aggressive surgical or radiation procedures required to achieve comfort.

The actual variation of time-dependent enhanced quality will depend on a
multitude of factors, including—but not limited to—diagnosis, co-morbidity,
culture, personal values and family needs. Any decision to crunch numbers
in this way must be accompanied by an obligation to determine how these
variables might influence the rate of quality enhancement. In general, it is
likely that cognitive integrity, lack of symptom distress and a robust support
network will favor heightened valuation, while cognitive disintegration, suffering and isolation will tend to mitigate the valuation effect. However, this
calculus is highly nuanced, in that health care providers often infer great
suffering and poor quality of life based on functional limitations and disability.[11] Therapeutic nihilism can easily undermine the ability to see value
beyond cure-oriented disease modification. On the other hand, palliative
care must embrace a perspective as broad as the notion of quality of life itself.

While this mathematical approach may strike some as highly reduction-
istic, such is the nature of cost effectiveness analysis. Applying the VIP treatment, so to speak, to patients near the end of life provides a means of ascribing
value to the multitude of things that take place when life is drawing to a close.
The VIP does not justify wasteful spending on measures that are inconsistent
with quality palliative care, i.e., those that do not target improved quality of
life for dying patients and their families. Health care economists, health care
authorities, and health care administrators rarely speak the language of existential growth, family reconciliation or societal morality. While introducing

the concept of VIP is unlikely to make them conversant in these areas, it does force the acknowledgment that these things have value and must be taken into account when considering end-of-life care budgets and resource allocation. How much value you ask? There, I'm afraid, the answer will always be relative.

References

1. Haycox H. Optimizing decision making and resource allocation in palliative care. *J Pain Symptom Manage.* 2009;38:45–53.
2. Lenert LA, Treadwell JR, Schwartz CE. Associations between health status and utilities implications for policy. *Med Care.* 1999;37:479–489.
3. Philipson T, Becker G, Goldman D, Murphy K. Terminal care and the value of life near its end. MFI Working Paper Series No. 2010-005. 2010. http://ssrn.com/abstract.1544510 (accessed September 15, 2010).
4. Ehrlich I. A model of the demand for longevity and the value of life extension. *J Polit Econ.* 1990;98:761–782.
5. Menec V, Lix L, Steinbach C, et al. *Patterns of Health Care Use and Cost at the End of Life.* Manitoba Centre for Health Policy; 2004.
6. Normand C. Measuring outcomes in palliative care: limitations of QALYs and the road to PalYs. *J Pain Symptom Manage.* 2009;38:27–31.
7. Zhang B, Wright AA, Huskamp HA, et al. Health care costs in the last week of life: associations with end-of-life conversations. *Arch Intern Med.* 2009;169:480–488.
8. Wright AA, Zhang B, Ray A, et al. Associations between end-of-life discussions, patient mental health, medical care near death, and caregiver bereavement adjustment. *JAMA.* 2008;300:1665–1673.
9. Morrison RS, Penrod JD, Cassel JB, et al. Palliative Care Leadership Centers' Outcomes Group. Cost savings associated with US hospital palliative care consultation programs. *Arch Intern Med.* 2008;168:1783–1790.
10. World Health Organization. WHO definition of palliative care. http://www.who.int/can cer/palliative/definition/en (accessed December 24, 2010).
11. Stienstra D, Chochinov HM. Vulnerability, disability, and palliative end-of-life care. *J Palliat Care.* 2006;22:166–174.

24

Vicarious Grief and Response to Global Disasters

This article offers a global perspective on an issue individual clinicians grapple with regularly; that is, what moves us to feel for another person's suffering? I recall being asked to see a mother of two young children who was receiving treatment for metastatic cancer on an inpatient oncology unit. The nurse requesting this consultation described the patient as "difficult," "challenging," and "hard to get along with." While the details of the case have faded over the years, I remember the patient giving me none of those impressions. As the referring nurse and I discussed the case, I discovered she and the patient were around the same age, as were their children. Upon reflection, this nurse recognized that being with this patient felt like looking into a mirror reflecting her worst nightmare. Irritation and withdrawal were her defensive, self-protective fallback.

Most clinicians know not all patients elicit the same feelings of connectedness. This usually depends on emotional chemistry, combining elements of disposition, aptitude, and imagination. By nature, are you wired to help others? Do you have the skills to make a difference? And can you imagine yourself or someone you love being in a similar situation? Chemical reactions can have more than one valence. This means that while a connection infused with caring and compassion can emerge, so too can the inclination to recoil or withdraw based on several factors worth exploring.

The first hurdle regarding connectedness is reconciling its place in the provision of healthcare. Contemporary medicine increasingly emphasizes biological and technical facets of patient care, what I refer to as the "transactional," given their focus on things we do to patients like tests and empirically based interventions. While these are critically important, we do ourselves, our patients, and their families a disservice when we neglect the relational aspects of medicine. Patients won't trust us in the absence of connectedness; they will be less revealing of their needs, leading to discordance in goals of care. As the article in Chapter 22 *stated, "Patients Are People*

In Search of Dignity. Harvey Max Chochinov, Oxford University Press. © Oxford University Press 2025.
DOI: 10.1093/9780197805145.003.0024

with Feelings That Matter," which is why relational elements of medicine are vital. Many of these messages were highlighted in my remarks to the incoming medical students at their White Coat Ceremony (see Chapter 37*).*

People often cite lack of time as a reason for limited engagement. When time is scarce, it is important to use it wisely and mindfully; that is, to be fully present, undistracted, and entirely focused on the patient. It is possible within the same few minutes to make a good or a bad impression. Studies have shown that the simple act of sitting rather than standing at the patient's bedside can expand their perception of how much time was spent and can significantly improve their satisfaction with the clinical encounter.

*Another explanation for "negative valence" reactions is avoidance of therapeutic helplessness. When our research group developed the Patient Dignity Inventory (*J Pain Symptom Manage. *2008;36:559–571), we included physical and psychological items, along with others that are existential and spiritual in nature. The latter include, for example, "feeling like I am no longer who I was," "feeling that I am a burden to others," "feeling I don't have control over my life," and "not being able to accept the way things are." Admittedly, these things are not easily or readily fixed. Despite that, clinicians must appreciate the potency of Intensive Caring (*Chapters 19 and 20*) and how showing up for patients— listening to what they are going through—is profound and inherently therapeutic.*

There are instances, such as illustrated by the prior case, where a negative valence yields emotional withdrawal in the service of self-protection. This coping mechanism becomes problematic, however, when it interferes with optimal person-centered care. As my former colleague Dr. Mike Harlos used to say, "If you intend to work in the kitchen, be prepared to get close enough to feel some heat, but not so close as to get burnt." In other words, empathic connection is a mindful dance choreographed within each clinical encounter. Proximity yields to distance and distance to proximity, based on the specifics of the clinical moment and the ephemeral chemistry between patient and healthcare provider.

Vicarious Grief and Response to Global Disasters. Harvey Max Chochinov. *The Lancet*, 2005;366:697–698. Reprinted with permission from Elsevier.

What shapes our response to global disasters? Most of what we know about grief comes from studies that track individual reactions to personal loss.[1] These studies mainly identify characteristics of bereavement and how it changes over time. Events, such as the tsunami at the end of last year in southern Asia, evoke a worldwide response whose phenomenology is not nearly as well understood. Whilst several investigators have examined psychological impairments in those directly affected, less is known about the nature of post-disaster vicarious grief within the broader global community.[2-5]

Disasters that evoke widespread response have several notable features, beginning with global visibility. The likelihood of vicarious grieving is proportionate to what the disaster literature describes as indirect or secondary exposure to coverage in the mass media.[3] Exposure to details about the disaster increases the likelihood of being preoccupied with intrusive thoughts about victims, and post-disaster distress.[3,4]

The Asian tsunami was marked by sudden, unanticipated, random, and numerous deaths—characteristics associated with lingering and pronounced grief reactions.

Other factors related to protracted grieving include multiple violent deaths, or deaths involving mutilation, such as the 9/11 terrorist attacks in the USA.[6,7] The very nature of these dramatic events disrupts our collective sense of stability and predictability, resulting in what some have described as a "shattering of the assumptive world."[7] This disruption of psychological homoeostasis can influence individual or community reactions, evoking fear, anxiety, vulnerability, and ultimately, a sense of feeling less safe.

Identification with the victim is another powerful mediator of response, predisposing to disaster-focused distress. After 9/11, vicarious victims were described as those who perceived real or imagined similarity to actual victims; they identified with victim experiences, despite being physically removed from the scene of the falling towers or having no direct connection with any of the victims.[5] This sense of identification appears to be connected to the disaster setting itself. It is easy to imagine being in an office tower, airplane, or on a beach; it is perhaps the ordinariness or imaginability of these pre-disaster settings that heightens identification with actual victims.[8]

How does vicarious grief compare between dramatic catastrophic events and chronic human disasters that are experienced daily around the world? Because of their chronicity, and despite their enormity, tragedies such as AIDS, malaria, and tuberculosis do not seem to resonate at an individual level in the same way as sudden dramatic catastrophes. AIDS kills more than

8000 people a day or one person every 10 s.[9] In 2004, WHO reported over 3 million deaths from AIDS, including 500,000 children under the age of 15 years.[9] An estimated 1.7 million people died from tuberculosis in 2003, including nearly 20% co-infected with HIV.[10]

Malaria accounts for 1–2 million deaths annually, claiming the life of an African child every 30 s.[11] In total, about 6 million people die of AIDS, tuberculosis, and malaria each year—over 16,000 preventable deaths a day.[12] Yet, ubiquitous chronic tragedies do not seem to move people in the same way as those that are sudden or dramatic.

Besides the acute and intense media attention the latter receive, there is the issue of imagination. Whilst most westerners can readily evoke images of sudden disasters, the prospect of dying from a chronic illness in the sub-Sahara lies beyond imagination.

Another aspect of post-disaster vicarious grief is lending or giving aid. Giving money or blood can help alleviate disaster-focused stress and establishes a sense of cohesion with a community joined in tragedy.[13] Patterns of philanthropy, however, appear to support the distinction between imaginable versus unimaginable disaster scenarios. For instance, Giving USA estimates that by the end of 2001, US$1.88 billion was received by the major relief funds for 9/11.[14] To date, international donors have pledged more than $5 billion towards tsunami relief.[8] Contrast this with the $200–300 million a year that the world spends on malarial control, or the $1.2 billion total funding available for tuberculosis control in the high-burden countries.[12] The annual funds spent on programmes for HIV/AIDS prevention, care, and support in low-income and middle-income countries are $1.8 billion.[15] The UN estimates that these countries would need $7–10 billion annually to mount a successful programme against the AIDS epidemic—according to the UN Secretary General, this sum represents 1% of the world's yearly military spending.[15]

A better understanding of post-disaster vicarious grief is important, because the psychology affecting individual reactions may guide community or global responses.

Understanding vicarious grief has public-health and public policy implications, because how we perceive and process these losses might partly influence how resources are allocated. Whilst abject poverty, disease, or persistent environmental crisis may not capture headlines or resonate in the same way as the more dramatic calamities, they are the chronic and hideous silent tsunamis of our time.

References

1. Parkes C. *Bereavement: Studies of Grief in Adult Life.* 3rd ed. Taylor & Francis; 2001.
2. Rubonis AV, Bickman L. Psychological impairment in the wake of disaster: the disaster-psychopathology relationship. *Psychol Bull.* 1991;109:384–399.
3. Silver RC, Holman EA, McIntosh DN, et al. Nationwide longitudinal study of psychological responses to September 11. *JAMA.* 2002;288:1235–1244.
4. Schlenger WE, Caddell JM, Ebert L, et al. Psychological reactions to terrorist attacks: findings from the National Study of Americans' Reactions to September 11. *JAMA.* 2002;288:581–588.
5. Wayment HA. It could have been me: vicarious victims and disaster focused distress. *Pers Soc Psychol Bull.* 2004;30:515–528.
6. Rando T. Vicarious bereavement. In: Strack S, ed. *Death and the Quest for Meaning.* Jason Aronson; 1997:257–274.
7. Rando T. Complications in mourning traumatic death. In: Corless I, Germino B, Pittman M, eds. *Dying, Death and Bereavement: Theoretical Perspectives and Other Ways of Knowing.* Jones and Barlett Publishers; 1994:253–271.
8. Nolan S. Federal tsunami aid hits 425 million as cash woes hurt African AIDS fight. *Globe and Mail* Jan. 11, 2005:A 1.
9. World Health Organization Regional Office for South-East Asia. HIV/AIDS: facts and figures, March 17, 2005. http://w3.whosea.org/EN/Section10/Section18/Section348.htm (accessed May 5, 2005).
10. World Health Organization. Global tuberculosis control—surveillance, planning, financing, 2005. www.who.int/tb/publications/global_report/2005/summary/en/index.html (accessed May 6, 2005).
11. World Health Organization. Malaria is alive and well and killing more than 3000 African children every day, April 25, 2003. http://www.who.int/mediacentre/news/releases/2003/pr33/en (accessed May 5, 2005).
12. Global Fund to Fight AIDS, Tuberculosis and Malaria. HIV/AIDS, tuberculosis and malaria: the status and impact of the three diseases, 2005. www.theglobalfund.org/en/files/about/replenishment/disease_report_en.pdf (accessed May 3, 2005).
13. Schuster MA, Stein BD, Jaycox L, et al. A national survey of stress reactions after the September 11, 2001, terrorist attacks. *N Engl J Med.* 2001;345:1507–1512.
14. American Association of Fundraising Counsel (AAFRC) Trust for Philanthropy. Charitable giving reaches $212 billion (Giving USA 2002, The Annual Report on Philanthropy for the Year 2001), June 20, 2002. http://www.aafrc.org/press_releases/trustreleases/charitablegiving.html (accessed May 5, 2005).
15. Alagiri P, Collins C, Summers T, et al. Global spending on HIV/AIDS: tracking public and private investments in AIDS prevention, care and research, 2001. http://www.kaisernetwork.org/health_cast/uploaded_files/Global_Spending.pdf (accessed May 6, 2005).

SECTION 4

REFLECTIONS ON HASTENING DEATH

25

In Praise of Wisdom

A Morality Tale

Despite how much I've published on the topic of death hastening, I do so with little pleasure. I'm most apt to put "pen to pad" (antiquated metaphor) when I feel annoyed or upset about something I've read or heard about medical assistance in dying (MAiD) or get what I would describe as an intellectual itch. Sometimes it's both.

Take the recent deliberations in the United Kingdom and the British Parliament passing legislation to allow for MAiD. On the eve of this pivotal vote, Conservative Member of Parliament Kit Malthouse said, "The death bed for far too many is a place of misery, torture and degradation, a rain of blood and vomit and tears." He added, "Please be clear that, whatever happens today, terminal people will still take their own lives. All we are deciding today is how." This is the sort of rhetoric and misinformation that moves me to want to set the record straight. With all due respect to Minister Malthouse, this does not describe normal dying but rather sounds like the hellscape of a Stephen King horror novel. But there is no process of fact checking or a "time out" to alert parliamentarians that they are being duped and that their "yea" vote has been manipulated by way of fear and a distorted picture of normal dying.

I recall some MAiD proponents declaring that the goal of the MAID provider, similar to the palliative care professional, is not to hasten death, but to support choice. This feels a bit like saying cardiac bypass surgery is not about saving lives but improving myocardial perfusion. It's doublespeak, smoke and mirrors, intended to distract, to bamboozle, and, for anyone with misgivings, to wear down resistance. It's exhausting, to say the least.

When I was asked to chair the External Panel for the Federal Government examining national and international perspectives on death-hastening practices, proponents were concerned that I would be biased and that the committee would deliver a report skewed in favor of restrictions and prohibitions, while not considering alternative perspectives. Over the

In Search of Dignity. Harvey Max Chochinov, Oxford University Press. © Oxford University Press 2025.
DOI: 10.1093/9780197805145.003.0025

course of our work, we received and considered 321 written submissions from civil-society organizations, academics, and individual citizens. We also held meetings with 73 individual experts in Canada, the United States, the Netherlands, Belgium, and Switzerland and consulted directly with 92 representatives of interveners, medical authorities, and stakeholders from 46 Canadian organizations. Despite widely diverse perspectives—from Dying with Dignity Canada to the Catholic Health Alliance of Canada— everyone appearing before our panel was treated with respect, and we provided a platform that allowed them to share their position with a panel keen to listen and to learn.

The same, unfortunately, cannot be said of some members of Canada's parliament and Senate, who were utterly closed-minded in considering perspectives other than their own. During various official hearings on MAiD, these individuals tried to dismiss and discredit and showed disdain toward witnesses whose testimony was at odds with their own firmly held beliefs. While these politicians are no doubt intelligent people, they failed to show wisdom—hence the annoyance and intellectual itch resulting in this article.

In Praise of Wisdom: A Morality Tale. Harvey Max Chochinov. *Journal of Palliative Medicine*, 2022;25(10);1460–1461. Reprinted with permission from Mary Ann Liebert, Inc.

Abstract
Wisdom and intelligence work best in unison. What happens, however, when seemingly smart people fail to exercise wisdom, either in social discourse, clinical encounters, or even within the broader political arena? This morality tale, in which Wisdom and Smart take each other on in a debate at a local bar, illustrates the fallout when these two are not on the same page.

Introducing the Cast

Medicine is fraught with controversy, particularly when engaging issues wherein life and death hang in the balance. In those instances, being smart allows one to sift through the complexity of information that may have a bearing on how things will play out. But intelligence alone is often insufficient. Lack of wisdom may see us arrive at solutions that are arguably right, but do not feel right; or can be justified, but do not feel just. With your indulgence, I have asked *Smart* and *Wisdom* to take part in this morality tale. I suspect they will explain this far better than I can.

Smart talks. Wisdom listens. Smart tends to be loud, whereas Wisdom is soft spoken. Smart always has answers. Wisdom tries hard to understand the questions. Smart moves quickly, whereas Wisdom takes its time. Smart can be bold and flashy. Wisdom is more subdued and humble. Smart always has something to say, whereas Wisdom knows that silence is sometimes the best response.

There is something incredibly attractive, even seductive, about Smart. Smart thinks quickly on its feet, always has a comeback and can nail a sound bite. Smart plays well on social media; Wisdom, not so much. Smart draws attention to itself and makes convincing pronouncements. Listening to Smart, things seem straightforward and black or white. People looking for simple solutions to difficult questions—in social situations, clinical encounters, or within the broader political arena—gravitate toward Smart.

Wisdom is contemplative. Wisdom tends to accumulate over time and with life experience. Wisdom looks for subtleties, nuances, and is not fooled by seemingly simple solutions to complex problems. Wisdom is patient, knows that time is not static and is ever moving forward into a future that often brings clarity, understanding, and even resolution. When they can work together, Wisdom adores hanging out with Smart, knowing that they are an inspiring duo. But when Smart and Wisdom are not on the same page, Wisdom knows that nothing good can come of it.

A Morality Tale

Smart and Wisdom walk into a bar. Smart orders a special brand of single malt whiskey, knowing it to be the perfect balance between quality and value. Since it is the middle of the day, and both must drive back to work, Wisdom settles for a Diet Coke. No sooner are they seated, when Smart decides to challenge Wisdom to a debate on whose defining characteristic is more important. Wisdom asks where this need to compete comes from and why such a debate is even necessary. Smart persists and begins to regale Wisdom on the virtues of being Smart. As Smart starts to talk louder, other bar patrons begin to take notice.

The crowd feels an immediate attraction to Smart, given it has shown up wearing an Armani suit and shiny black leather Hugo Boss shoes. Wisdom on the other hand is wearing a frumpy woollen cardigan, sweatpants, and Birkenstocks. Struggling to get a word in edgewise, Wisdom tries to impress on Smart that they work best together:

> *"Smart without Wisdom is like Yin without Yang; like a fancy car without an engine; or like having a full tank of gas but nowhere to go."*

Smart does not really have a good comeback, and so, suddenly jumps on top of one of the bar tables, shouting, "Smart can't be broken! Wise Cracks!"

The room goes wild! Everybody loves it, although no one knows quite what it means. Wisdom can immediately sense the tide has turned, as Smart whips the crowd into a frenzy, while the room throbs to their chant, "Wise Cracks, Wise Cracks, Wise Cracks!" Wisdom slinks off into a corner, while Smart basks in the glow of victory and is plied with free drinks from patrons, raising numerous toasts to just how clever Smart has been.

Epilogue

On the drive back to work in its BMW, Smart is in a motor vehicle accident in which two pedestrians are seriously injured. A blood alcohol test taken at the scene exceeds the legal limit. A court date is pending.

Wisdom stays on a while longer at the bar, largely ignored, sipping on what remains of its Diet Coke. Wisdom finally exits to no fanfare whatsoever, contemplating *what does all of this really mean and is there some bigger lesson to be learned?* Wisdom then drives its Volvo, always just ever so slightly below the speed limit, arriving back at work safe and sound.

Conclusion

The inspiration to write this piece came in the context of observing and taking part in national discussions regarding medical assistance in dying. Like so many divisive issues, people seem to be more interested in racking up points than they are in listening, reflecting, and being open to opinions and evidence that might challenge their worldview. Being smart, sheer intelligence, does not seem to confer immunity from this troubling inclination. Which is why, whether considering clinical work, setting health care policy, or deliberating broader political issues, I find myself compelled to write in praise of Wisdom.

26

Secobarbital in Seattle

Why Lose Sleep?

Shortly after launching its assisted suicide program, the Seattle Cancer Care Alliance published an article stating they did not post information about death-with-dignity legislation or their services in public spaces. This demonstrates awareness of the impact this information might have on patients and families. Providing a death-hastening option asserts that it is a viable alternative. This communication is by no means emotionally or spiritually neutral, since it affirms ending your life under these circumstances is a reasonable consideration. It also says that as your healthcare provider, I am prepared to accede to your request.

What we do and say to patients matters. So too is our way of being with patients and our attitude toward them. The pressure to find solutions to difficult problems often elicits a "doing to" rather than "being with" response; I think of this as the distinction between transactional (things we do to patients) versus relational (ways of being with patients) facets of healthcare.

I recently met a woman living with advanced cancer who had applied and been approved for medical assistance in dying (MAiD). Her story was one of lifelong disappointments and relationships that never seemed to work out as she'd hoped. She eventually came to see herself as flawed and undesirable. Others didn't seem to like her, she told me, and she wasn't sure she liked herself. When she became ill, MAiD seemed like a perfect and convenient way out. But weeks had passed since the MAiD team had signed off on her application, leading me to ask her, "Why aren't you dead?" She rather sheepishly explained that her palliative care nurses were all very nice and seemed to genuinely enjoy her company, so, for now, she was content to carry on.

Her story underscores the importance of "being with" and how it affirms a patient's sense of worth and sustains hope. (The chapter on Intensive Caring [Chapter 19] offers evidence for how the relationship between patients and healthcare professionals can moderate suicidality in patients who are

In Search of Dignity. Harvey Max Chochinov, Oxford University Press. © Oxford University Press 2025.
DOI: 10.1093/9780197805145.003.0026

severely ill.) For the most part, hope is affiliated with expectations for what is yet to come. In the context of life-limiting illness, hope takes on interesting new textures as it becomes uncoupled from expectations for time and takes up residency within the realm of meaning and hope. Those can be found by way of connectedness and being in the moment—in the "here now." This is what makes "being with" such a potent response to human suffering, for families (see Chapter 20*) and healthcare providers alike.*

Secobarbital in Seattle: Why Lose Sleep? Harvey Max Chochinov *Nature Reviews Clinical Oncology*, 2013;10:369–370. Reprinted with permission from Nature Portfolio.

About 2 years ago, the Seattle Cancer Care Alliance (SCCA) added physician-assisted suicide to their list of offerings for terminally ill patients thought to be within 6 months of death. A recent publication in the *New England Journal of Medicine*[1] describes how this service, sanctioned under the Washington Death with Dignity Act, has turned out. Although the report includes all the expected metrics—how many people inquired into the Death with Dignity Program, how many received a lethal prescription of secobarbital, how many died because of said prescription—the authors' take-home message is that the program has been well accepted by patients and clinicians, and that the business of medicine at SCCA goes on as usual. So, why lose sleep?

According to Greek mythology, a Chimera was a monstrous fire-breathing creature, usually depicted as a lion, with the head of a goat arising from its back and a tail that ended in a snake's head. Describing such a creature depends completely on where one stands; based on their vantage point, observers might conceivably recount accurate and yet entirely contradictory images. Clearly, the issue of physician-assisted suicide and euthanasia is a modern-day Chimera, and it remains amongst the most polarizing and contentious issues in all of medicine. Legions of opponents and proponents have waged battle, armed with powerful and seemingly convincing arguments: autonomy, the sanctity of life, the right to die, the slippery slope, the imperative of palliative care, the integrity of medicine as we know it and, lest we forget, dignity. And yet, we seem no closer to resolving how to tame this beast; as my daughter, who studies medieval literature, tells me, "slaying dragons is a tricky business" (L. J. Chochinov, personal communication).

It seems futile to rehash all the same arguments, and hubris to think that one more voice, on either side of the political/legal/ethical/clinical fence, could make any real difference. Although the report[1] suggests that there is no need to lose sleep, I find myself unable to rest easy. For instance, we are told that of 200 surveyed SCCA physicians, 29 respondents identified themselves as willing to consult and prescribe for the Death with Dignity Program. Aside from their willingness to be involved with the program, nothing is said about their expertise in attending to the needs of dying patients. Given that a desire for death and requests for assisted dying are usually driven by psychosocial and existential considerations,[2,3] it is important to know what level of expertise these physicians have in those matters. Prior studies on health-care provider willingness to offer assisted suicide demonstrate an association with various personal factors including diminished empathy and lesser knowledge of symptom management; in fact, it would seem that doctors who have least contact with patients with a terminal disease are most likely to support legalization of assisted suicide, while those with the most experience are oppositely inclined.[4–6]

The Death with Dignity Program describes a prominent role for designated social worker patient advocates.[1] Advocacy consists of confirming that a terminal prognosis has been documented, arranging for a prescribing physician, documentation of the patient's wish for physician-assisted dying, verifying that the patient is a Washington resident and, most critical, the completion of a psychosocial assessment—that is, evaluating patients for depression and decision-making capacity. Although the report is silent on the characteristics of these social workers,[1] prior studies examining the role of mental health professionals in hastened death decisions are telling. A study of psychiatrists in Oregon found that those opposed to assisted suicide were more likely to work with the patient to prevent the suicide, whereas those who supported it were more likely to either take no further action or support the patient in obtaining a lethal prescription.[7] The authors conclude that, "[psychiatrists'] moral beliefs influence how they might evaluate a patient requesting assisted suicide." Only 6% of psychiatrists were very confident that they could adequately assess whether a psychiatric disorder was impairing the judgment of a patient requesting assisted suicide within a single session; just over half felt very confident that they could do so within the context of a long-term relationship.[7] What implications does this have for health-care providers and consultants who are neither mental health experts, nor necessarily know patients for any extended period of time?

Loggers *et al.*[1] indicate that no one given a lethal prescription required a mental health evaluation for depression or decisional incapacity; in fact, Death with Dignity participants were infrequently referred to the pain or palliative care services. Why might that be? The authors report that it was because of an absence of symptoms (such as depression or questions regarding decisional capacity) at the time of the request to be part of the program. It would seem then, that symptoms that are indicative of suffering, such as losing autonomy, loss of dignity, feeling a burden to others (all prominent amongst the beneficiaries of the Death with Dignity Program), are not on the therapeutic radar, or perhaps deemed beyond the purview or reach of medicine.

"Death with dignity" has become a global euphemism for physician-assisted suicide and euthanasia. That these measures are so universally affiliated with the language of dignity is surely an indictment of the culture of medicine, which largely ignores death and tends to abandon patients when cure is no longer viable. This culture of medicine often fails to deliver adequate relief from pain and distress associated with terminal illness, despite there being effective means to do so (it is worse for dying children than adults; worse for the frail elderly and cognitively impaired; worse for people who are poor, members of ethnic minorities or the disabled; worse for people with non-cancer-related fatal illnesses; and worse for people living in rural or remote regions).[8] When lethal prescriptions and fatal injections are hailed as "death with dignity," it underscores how few expectations patients have of medicine, and its ability to offer effective, humane alternatives.

Dignity conserving palliative care requires thoughtful attention to patients' physical, psychological, existential and spiritual dimensions of suffering.[9] It requires that personhood not be overshadowed by patienthood. When our research group published a dignity-conserving approach to end of life care,[10] Faye Girth, the executive director of the Hemlock Society USA (which was a national right-to-die organization) conceded "if most individuals with terminal illness were treated this way, the incentive to end their lives would be greatly reduced."[10] To be clear, palliative care should no more be seen as the perfect foil to suffering, than medicine should be pitched as the perfect foil to death. There will always be a tiny minority of patients who, despite the best care possible, will want to control the timing and circumstances of their death; and will want the law of the land changed to ensure their physicians can help them do so. One thing is for certain—this Chimera will not be easily slain.

References

1. Loggers ET, Starks H, Shannon-Dudley M, et al. Implementing a Death with Dignity program at a comprehensive cancer center. *N Engl J Med.* 2013;368: 1417–1424.
2. Wilson KG, Chochinov HM, McPherson CJ, et al. Desire for euthanasia or physician-assisted suicide in palliative cancer care. *Health Psychol.* 2007;26: 314–323.
3. Chochinov HM, Wilson KG, Enns M, et al. Desire for death in the terminally ill. *Am J Psychiatry.* 1995;152: 1185–1191.
4. Portenoy RK, Coyle N, Kash KM, et al. Determinants of the willingness to endorse assisted suicide: a survey of physicians, nurses and social workers. *Psychosomatics.* 1997;38: 277–287.
5. Bachman JG, Alcser KH, Doukas DJ, et al. Attitudes of Michigan physicians and the public toward legalizing physician-assisted suicide and voluntary euthanasia. *N Engl J Med.* 1996;334: 303–309.
6. Cohen JS, Fihn SD, Boyko EJ, et al. Attitudes toward assisted suicide and euthanasia among physicians in Washington State. *N Engl J Med.* 1994; 331: 89–94.
7. Ganzini L, Fenn DS, Lee MA, et al. Attitudes of Oregon psychiatrists toward physician-assisted suicide. *Am J Psychiatry.* 1996;153: 1469–1475.
8. Hughes A. Poor, homeless, and underserved populations. In: Ferrell B, Coyle N, eds. *Oxford Textbook of Palliative Nursing.* 3rd ed. Oxford University Press; 2010:745–755.
9. Chochinov HM. Dignity-conserving care—a new model for palliative care: helping the patient feel valued. *JAMA.* 2002; 287: 2253–2260.
10. Girth F. Dignity-conserving care at the end of life. *JAMA* 2002;288: 162.

27

Canada Failing on Palliative Care

The years have flown by since the publication of this article in 2015. So many things were about to happen that couldn't have been anticipated or even imagined. In a unanimous decision on February 6, 2015, the Supreme Court overturned the criminal code provisions prohibiting physician-assisted death for eligible patients, giving mentally competent Canadian adults with enduring, intolerable suffering the right to a doctor's assistance in dying. The rationale for the court's decision has always struck me as a circuitous bit of logic. The court ruled that sections 14 (which prohibits a person from consenting to their own death) and 241(b) (which prohibits assisting suicide) of the Criminal Code were unconstitutional, in violation of the right to life, liberty, and security of the person under the Canadian Charter of Rights and Freedoms. In other words, not being able to access hastened death might cause someone to take their life earlier while still able to, rather than waiting and possibly losing their ability to do so later. Thus, the court ruled, your right to death protects your right to life. Extraordinary but true, nevertheless.

Following the court's decision, the government needed to sort out its response. I was appointed chair of the External Panel on Options for a Legislative Response to Carter v. Canada, established by the government of Prime Minister Steven Harper. Shortly thereafter, the government fell and the Trudeau liberals took power. Despite that, our mandate was renewed and our work continued, with the final report released January 18, 2016. After much debate and various committees weighing in on this singularly contentious issue, Bill C-14, also known as the Medical Assistance in Dying (MAiD) bill, was introduced in the Canadian House of Commons on April 14, 2016, by the Minister of Justice, Jody Wilson-Raybould. It received Royal Assent on June 17, 2016.

The initial bill showed some restraint, limiting eligibility to those with "a reasonably foreseeable death." At the time, this seemed like an important guardrail, limiting MAiD to patients trying to escape what they anticipated would be a horrible death. Who could know the alchemy of autonomy and

In Search of Dignity. Harvey Max Chochinov, Oxford University Press. © Oxford University Press 2025.
DOI: 10.1093/9780197805145.003.0027

fear behaves like helium, taking up as much space as possible? Helium, being helium, can't be contained. On September 11, 2019, the Superior Court of Quebec declared restricting euthanasia to those whose death is reasonably foreseeable violated the Charter's guarantee to "life, liberty, and security of the person" as well as the Charter's guarantee of "equal protection" under the law. The reasonably foreseeable clause in the federal euthanasia legislation was declared unconstitutional. The federal government chose not to appeal this decision. In March 2021, legislation was amended by Bill C-7 allowing MAiD for those suffering from a grievous and irremediable condition when death was not reasonably foreseeable. A last-minute amendment from the Senate of Canada introduced a sunset clause, allowing MAiD for those whose sole underlying medical condition is a mental illness. This was to have come into effect in March 2023. It was then delayed by 1 year to March 2024, and further pushed back to March 2027. Further expansions being contemplated include advance directives (now available under Quebec legislation) and mature minors.

Who could have predicted more than 60,000 MAiD deaths since the introduction of legislation in 2016, accounting for 4.7% of all deaths in Canada? But then again, helium being helium, I suppose we should have seen it coming.

Canada Failing on Palliative Care by Harvey Max Chochinov. An earlier version of this essay first appeared in *Toronto Star* on February 18, 2015.

A few days after the Supreme Court of Canada overturned the prohibition against doctor-assisted suicide, I received a note from a wonderful colleague of mine saying that her closest friend's 53-year-old son had just died of spinal cancer. Two weeks before his death he had visited his general practitioner, experiencing "terrible pain." Despite his anguish, his physician refused to give him morphine, claiming that because he was a smoker, he was "more likely to become addicted."

While this seems unfathomable, even grotesque, ignorance and lack of skill in attending to the needs of dying patients are still tragically common in Canada.

Despite the impressive strides that palliative care has taken—in areas such as pain and symptom management, and sensitivities to the psychosocial, existential, and spiritual challenges facing dying patients and their families—at their time of licensure, physicians have been taught less about pain management than those graduating from veterinary medicine. Once in practice, most physicians have knowledge deficiencies that can significantly impair their ability to manage cancer pain.

Doctors are also not generally well-trained to engage in end-of-life conversations, meaning that goals of care often remain unclear; and patients may not receive the care they want or the opportunity to live out their final days in the place they would want to die.

In light of the Supreme Court's decision, these issues have never been more important, nor the need to resolve them ever more pressing. The court has given Parliament a year to sort out how it will move forward and rewrite the Criminal Code. Within these deliberations, it should be noted that the authority to provide a hastened death will be conferred on physicians, many of whom lack core competencies to care for patients nearing death.

To be clear, dying badly in Canada will rarely be the fallout of not having access to a lethal overdose or injection, and will almost invariably be the result of inadequate or substandard end-of-life care. With the clock ticking, now is the time for physicians to learn how to look after their patients until the very end.

The Supreme Court felt that patients needed to be provided with more choices. By adding doctor-assisted suicide into the mix, what options will dying patients in Canada actually have?

For 70 to 80 per cent of Canadians, palliative care is not available and hence, not a real choice. A dear friend of mine recently died of brain cancer. She spent her final months in hospice, where she received exquisite end-of-life care. She died comfortably and in as much peace as can be found by someone having to leave this world far too soon.

In the future, how might this kind of scenario play itself out in the many Canadian settings that do not have adequate palliative care? There, the choices will come down to settling for sub-optimal care; dislocating from friends and family to seek out better care elsewhere; or, if one is so inclined, considering medically hastened death.

We are about to become a country that extends patients the right to a hastened death but offers no legislative guarantees or assurances that they will be well looked after until they die.

As Canada deliberates its response to the court's decision, federal and provincial governments will need to make substantive investments in hospice and palliative care to offer patients and families choices that are equitable, compassionate, and real.

While autonomy has driven the "right to die" agenda, fear has been its engine. Now policymakers will need to grapple with how to draw a circle around autonomy, which means determining for whom and under what conditions medically hastened death will be permitted. Establishing those boundaries has implications for who will feel more or less afraid, who will feel more or less valued and who will anticipate death with more or less sense of calm.

Of this we can be sure: the width of that circle and the stability of its diameter will profoundly influence the culture of caring for dying Canadians, and those among us who are most vulnerable, for generations to come.

28

Medical Assistance in Dying

Data and Casting Assertions Aside

This article was written out of frustration. Everyone is entitled to their opinion; I'm good with that. And not everyone needs to always agree; again, that works for me. But when option is wrapped in partial or twisted data posing as fact, I find that infuriating. That's what happened during a symposium on medical assistance in dying (MAiD), when certain presenters— vocal proponents of medically assisted dying—engaged in that kind of sophistry.

I believe there are states of being worse than death. Trusted and experienced palliative care colleagues, who have taken care of thousands of patients over the course of their careers, tell me they can recall "a few" patients for whom hastened death might have been justified. But what happens when the law of the land makes that a real option? I remember long ago attending an international palliative care congress, listening to the late, wonderful professor of law Robert "Bo" Burt. He was part of a panel discussing Sue Rodriguez, whose request to die while living with amyotrophic lateral sclerosis went all the way to the Supreme Court of Canada. Bo dispensed with the usual arguments by asking the audience to assume she wasn't depressed, nor being coerced. He also asked us to imagine her care was optimal, despite persisting intolerable suffering. "Let's assume," he said, "that hastened death is what she wanted, and she felt in her best interest." He then asked us to consider the fallout of legislation that would accommodate her request. While some details have faded, the essence of his argument was that while death hastening might be rationalized for an individual, its viability unravels when contemplated as a social policy.

The Supreme Court of Canada stressed that MAiD should be a "stringently limited, carefully monitored system of exceptions." And then they placed the divine power of dispensing death in the hands of mere mortals. Little wonder the British Columbia Civil Liberties Association (BCCLA), which was on the forefront of the fight to decriminalize MAiD almost a

In Search of Dignity. Harvey Max Chochinov, Oxford University Press. © Oxford University Press 2025. DOI: 10.1093/9780197805145.003.0028

decade ago, is now calling on the provinces and federal governments to re-
view medically assisted dying legislation to ensure proper safeguards are
in place. The BCCLA stated there are "concerning reports" of people being
offered MAiD in circumstances that may not legally qualify or are the result
of intolerable social circumstances. This statement came after the family of a
52-year-old man who received MAiD while on a day pass from a Vancouver
psychiatric hospital launched a constitutional challenge to the procedure's
legal framework.

With the rate of MAiD in Quebec being higher than in most provinces, the
head of their commission on end-of-life care, which monitors MAiD in that
province, recently sparked headlines when he claimed that in Quebec "we're
now no longer dealing with an exceptional treatment, but a treatment that is
very frequent." As my dear friend and colleague Kathryn Mannix wrote, "Once
the euthanasia genie is out of the bottle, you must be careful what you wish for."

Medical Assistance in Dying: Data and Casting Assertions Aside. Harvey
Max Chochinov. *Journal of Palliative Medicine*, 2023;26(1):9–12. Reprinted
with permission from Mary Ann Liebert, Inc. publishers.

Abstract
Various assertions have been made regarding why eligibility for medical
assistance in dying (MAiD) should be expanded. Examining these and
the studies used to support them should clear the way for thoughtful data
monitoring and research into why some patients make death hastening
requests. This will not only improve MAiD practices in Canada, but will lead
to better more effective palliative care for patients whose suffering leads them
to covet death.

* * * * *

In 2015, I was appointed Chair of the Canadian Federal Government's
External Panel for a Legislative Response to *Carter versus Canada*.[1] Our
panel was tasked with reviewing all facets of euthanasia and assisted suicide, to help inform and guide parliamentarians in crafting new legislation. Our mandate included an environmental scan, gleaning lessons from
constituencies around the world already permitting some form of physician
hastened death. Six years later, the eyes of the world are now on Canada; eyes
that no doubt see how policies originally designed to assist dying patients

hasten their death have morphed into legislation that is no longer restricted to those nearing death, providing access to patients with incurable, although not imminently fatal illness, disease or disability, and starting in March 2023, those whose sole underlying medical condition is mental illness.

Some interesting arguments and rational for expanding MAiD in Canada were presented at a recent two-day symposium I attended entitled, Medical Assistance in Dying (MAiD) in Canada: A Multidisciplinary Pan-Canadian Knowledge Translation Initiative to Improve Practice Documents and Plan a Research Agenda on Suffering in the Context of a MAiD Request. This McGill University hosted pan-Canadian meeting, sponsored by the Canadian Institutes of Health Research and the Réseau québécois de recherche en soins palliatifs et de fin de vie, involved multiple clinicians and scientists in the field of MAiD, palliative care, and suicide prevention.

Other attendees included delegates from Health Canada, the Canadian Institute of Health Information, different professional associations, and government representatives. Having listened very closely to the proceedings, I come away with a deeper understanding of some assertions being made by those promoting expanded access to MAiD, and how data are used to support their position.

The first assertion of MAiD proponents is that MAiD is not driven by an inability to access palliative care. Although reference is made to the 2020 Health Canada Report on MAiD,[2] which indicates that 82.8% of MAiD recipients obtain palliative care services, there seems little concern that the only information collected about palliative care for MAiD recipients is whether it was received or not and for how long. These data, submitted by MAiD providers, are silent on what defines, and what minimal threshold constitutes "receiving palliative care." Imagine a patient who, after two years of eschewing health care for fear of being exposed to COVID-19, presents with widely metastatic cancer, associated with profound pain and suffering due to feeling a burden to his family, having received no supports whatsoever. A palliative care consultation recommends aggressive analgesia and supports for total pain, despite which he insists on having MAiD. Would such a patient be deemed a palliative care recipient, or more accurately, categorized as the epitome of failure to provide early and consistent palliation? Suffering, like cancer, grows, spreads, and if left unchecked, kills. The Health Canada report,[2] indicating 37.1% of MAiD patients receive palliative care for less than one month, and 54.8% greater than one month (with 8.1% unknown) offers insufficient data to affirm that these patients are being palliated in a manner designed to keep their suffering in check.

Another study intended to reinforce that MAiD has nothing to do with access to palliative care, reports the early experience of MAiD in Ontario, indicating that "palliative care providers were involved at any point in the care of 77.2% of patients, and at the time of the request for MAiD in 74.4%."[3] Similar to the Health Canada report,[2] this study reports the involvement of palliative care of any kind, without any specificity whatsoever of what that means. This is akin to reporting how many people took a drug, although neglecting to provide the dose, the route, and duration of administration.

Another observation made in support of this assertion is that patients with cancer, compared with those with organ failure or frailty, are far more likely to receive any palliative care, community-based palliative care, and do so for much longer periods of time.[4] Although this study says nothing about MAiD, it is used to argue that if the provision of MAiD was driven by limited access to palliative care or unmet palliative care needs, we simply would not see more than three times the rate of MAiD in cancer compared with noncancer illness. This fails to say that a predictable trajectory of advanced cancers means these patients are usually eligible for most palliative care services; and under Canada's original C-14 legislation—requiring a reasonably foreseeable death—meet eligibility criteria for MAiD. In contrast, clinicians often struggle or are reticent to prognosticate with confidence in non-malignant progressive life-limiting conditions; whereas patients with chronic noncancer conditions often have life expectancies that exceed reasonably foreseeable death. In other words, the lower uptake of MAiD in noncancer patients has little to do with their palliative care utilization, but rather, is likely because they are not, or are not identified as being, eligible.

A final argument regarding access to palliative care and MAiD observes that countries with the highest opioid utilization are those with the highest rates of MAiD. If availability of opioids, as a proxy for access to palliative care, averted the need for MAiD, proponents argue that the data ought to move in exactly the opposite direction. This fails to even scratch the surface of complexity regarding the international availability of opioids, the profound sociopolitical differences between developed and developing countries, and the global disparities in the organization, provision, and quality of health care.

Between 2011 and 2013, greater than 95% of global opioid analgesic use occurred in a small number of high-income countries, accounting for only

15% of the global population, whereas the use of opioid analgesics in other parts of the world is disproportionately low and does not meet the basic needs for pain control.[5] Latin America consumes <1% of the world's morphine.[6] Colombia is unique, in that despite limited access to opioids resulting from deficiencies in the procurement processes, insufficient human resources, excessive bureaucratic tasks, insufficient number of pharmacies authorized to dispense controlled medications, lack of training in health care professions, and overly restrictive laws and regulations governing opioid availability, assisted suicide and euthanasia were decriminalized for patients more than six years old.[6–8]

Colombia notwithstanding, countries with low access to opioids, for various complex geopolitical, cultural, economic, and historical reasons, have not legalized euthanasia or assisted suicide. In other words, the low uptake of death hastening options in developing countries has little to do with opioid availability, but rather, simply reflects these life-ending alternatives are not allowed.

The next assertion used to promote expanded access to MAiD is that requests are not primarily driven by physical suffering. This argument is meant to neutralize the potential influence palliative care might have in mitigating suffering that manifests as a wish to die. In other words, if palliative care can address physical suffering, and the latter is seen as a driver of requests for hastened death, MAiD would seem a less attractive option. Health Canada reports 57.6% of MAiD recipients have inadequate pain control (or concern), and 46% inadequate control of symptoms other than pain (or concern).[4] A study of Ontarians receiving MAiD reported 99.5% had physical suffering.[2] Along with minimizing the potential influence of physical suffering on MAiD, the case is made that palliative care has limited ability to offer relief.

For example, a study of family proxies is highlighted, reporting 47.5% of their decedents who received specialized palliative care services (SPCS) in the last two weeks of life were somewhat (20.4%) or very (27.1%) uncomfortable.[9] The study authors point out that people with more complex symptoms are more likely to be referred to SPCS, and that families tend to rate symptoms more severely than patients. Another study used to curb the promise of palliative care to deliver comfort illustrates high symptom burden toward death.[10] However, many of the prevalent symptoms reported in the study during the final seven days of life, such as loss of appetite, drowsiness, fatigue, sleep, urinary/fecal incontinence, dysphagia to solids and liquids, may represent not so much the limitations of palliative care, but the inevitable consequences of what happens to bodies as they are dying.[10]

It is also asserted that existential suffering is the most profound influence on requests for MAiD. Health Canada data indicate that loss of ability to engage in meaningful activities (86.3%) and loss of ability to perform activities of daily living (83.4%) are the most prominent sources of suffering for those receiving MAiD.[4] Although proponents characterize these as existential suffering, loss of the ability to engage in meaningful activities or activities of daily living implicates various and diverse challenges, including symptom distress, functional decline, and grief associated with diminished autonomy.

The Health Canada data delineating sources of suffering for patients receiving MAiD indicate that 3% experience emotional distress/anxiety/fear/existential suffering.[2] The typology of existential distress, such as fractured dignity, is complex, and requires a deep understanding of, and attentiveness to, physical, psychosocial, and spiritual assaults that can undermine personhood; this is fundamental to various approaches addressing existential suffering in patients nearing death.[11]

Having elevated the prominence of existential distress as a driver of MAiD, proponents assert that there is little to be done about this particular driver of a wish to die. One witness, supporting expanded MAiD eligibility, told the Special Joint Parliamentary Committee on MAiD that, "this is a type of suffering for which we have very little or nothing to offer."[12] Decades of research, clinical practice, and academic inquiry appear to have no standing in making this assertion.[13] Instead, the evidence used to support this argument includes a meta-analysis of randomized controlled trials of existential interventions on spiritual, psychological, and physical wellbeing in adult patients with cancer.[14]

Although some—trying to emphasize how little there is, aside from MAiD, to address existential suffering—have characterized the findings as unimpressive, the effect sizes for existential well-being (0.52), quality of life (0.21), hope (0.43), and self-efficacy (0.5) are not inconsiderable. The study authors conclude that their "analysis provides evidence that adult patients with cancer across all stages and types benefit from existential interventions,"[14] whereas the editors of the special issue this study appeared in conclude that this analysis demonstrates "clear benefits arise from existentially oriented psychotherapy."[15]

In the absence of targeted research and detailed data collection, assertions all too easily fill in the gap. Although there are widely differing opinions on MAiD, there are places we ought to find common ground.

1. The patient's voice must routinely be included in MAiD research and data monitoring.
2. We need a deeper understanding of what causes patients to want MAiD.
3. We need detailed data about psychosocial, supportive, palliative, existential, and spiritual measures that patients are offered and/or provided over the course of their condition leading to MAiD requests.
4. We must continue to develop and evaluate ways of addressing suffering that leads people to want to hasten death.

Health Canada states that, "federal public reporting on Medical Assistance in Dying continues to be a critical component to support transparency and foster public trust in the application of the law."[16] Although they acknowledge the need for the "consistent collection of information and public reporting,"[16] how can there be transparency or public trust when no patient-level data whatsoever are being gathered? Currently, the only data collected by the Government of Canada for patients receiving MAiD is a form that takes nine minutes, on average according to Health Canada, for MAiD providers to complete.[17] Surely understanding why patients want MAiD warrants more time than that. It is time to cast assertions aside; and instead, conduct research and gather data needed to fully understand requests for MAiD. This will not only improve MAiD practices in Canada but will enhance our ability to provide better and more effective palliative care for patients whose suffering leads them to covet death.

References

1. *Consultation on Physician-Assisted Dying: Summary of Results and Key Findings. Final Report.* December 15, 2015. https://www.justice.gc.ca/eng/rp-pr/other-autre/pad-amm/pad.pdf (last accessed October 12, 2022).
2. *Second Annual Report on Medical Assistance in Dying in Canada 2020.* https://www.canada.ca/en/health-canada/services/medical-assistance-dying/annualreport-2020.html (last accessed August 21, 2020).
3. Downar J, Fowler RA, Halko R, et al. Early experience with medical assistance in dying in Ontario, Canada: a cohort study. *CMAJ.* 2020;192(8):E173–E181.
4. Kendzerska T, Nickerson JW, Hsu AT, et al. End-of-life care in individuals with respiratory diseases: a population study comparing the dying experience between those with

chronic obstructive pulmonary disease and lung cancer. *Int J Chron Obstruct Pulmon Dis.* 2019;14:1691–1701.

5. Berterame S, Erthal J, Thomas J, et al. Use of and barriers to access to opioid analgesics: a worldwide, regional, and national study. *Lancet.* 2016;387:1644–1656.

6. Pain & Policy Studies Group. *Availability of Opioid Analgesics in Latin America and the World.* Prepared for 1st Congress of the Latin American Association of Palliative Care, 7th Latin American Course on Medicine and Palliative Care; March 20–22, 2002.

7. Leon MX, De Lima L, Florez S, et al. Improving availability of and access to opioids in Colombia: description and preliminary results of an action plan for the country. *J Pain Symptom Manage.* 2009;3:758–766.

8. World Federation Right to Die Societies. https://wfrtds.org/worldmap/colombia/ (last accessed July 31, 2022).

9. Currow DC, Ward AM, Plummer JL, et al. Comfort in the last 2 weeks of life: relationship to accessing palliative care services. *Support Care Cancer.* 2008;16:1255–1263.

10. Hui D, dos Santos R, Chisholm GB, et al. Symptom expression in the last seven days of life among cancer patients admitted to acute palliative care units. *J Pain Symptom Manage.* 2015;50:488–494.

11. Chochinov HM, Hassard T, McClement S, et al. The landscape of distress in the terminally ill. *J Pain Symptom Manage.* 2009;38:641–649.

12. AMAD Committee Meeting, Parliament of Canada. https://parl.ca/DocumentViewer/en/44-1/AMAD/meeting-4/evidence#Int-11644568 (last accessed August 21, 2022).

13. Chochinov HM, Breitbart W, eds. *The Handbook of Psychiatry in Palliative Medicine.* Oxford University Press; 2012.

14. Bauereiß N, Obermaier S, Özünal SE, et al. Effects of existential interventions on spiritual, psychological, and physical well-being in adult patients with cancer: systematic review and meta-analysis of randomized controlled trials. *Psychooncology.* 2018;27:2531–2545.

15. Vehling S, Kissane DW. Existential distress in cancer: alleviating suffering from fundamental loss and change. *Psychooncology.* 2018;27:2525–2530.

16. *Third Annual Report on Medical Assistance in Dying in Canada*; 2021. https://www.canada.ca/en/health-canada/services/medical-assistance-dying/annual-report-2021.html (last accessed August 21, 2020).

17. *Canada Gazette*, Part I, Volume 156, Number 21: Regulations Amending the Regulations for the Monitoring of Medical Assistance in Dying. https://canadagazette.gc.ca/rp-pr/p1/2022/2022-05-21/html/reg1-eng.html (last accessed August 21, 2022).

29

Protecting, Caring for the Mentally Ill

As the sunset clause allowing people with severe refractory mental illnesses to be eligible for medical assistance in dying (MAiD) was about to expire, I provided this testimony to the liberal caucus:

Parliamentarians must understand that denying access to MAiD for patients with mental illness is NOT discrimination. In 1950, during the Supreme Court case *Dennis v. United States*, Supreme Court Justice Felix Frankfurter said, "It was a wise man who said that there is no greater inequality than the equal treatment of unequals." Section 15 of the Charter makes it clear that every individual in Canada is to be treated with the same respect, dignity, and consideration. At the same time as it protects equality, the Charter also allows for certain laws or programs that aim to improve the conditions of disadvantaged individuals or groups.

While MAiD proponents argue that denial of MAiD for mental illness is discrimination and exceptionalism, the Charter recognizes that certain groups or individuals have exceptional needs and need to be treated as such. While the Charter says, "Every individual is equal before and under the law and has the right to the equal protection and equal benefit of the law without discrimination," equality does not mean everyone is to be treated the same.

We build seniors homes because we recognize the unique needs of the elderly; we create daycare centers because we appreciate the special needs of young children; we support the employment equity act, which states "employment equity means more than treating persons the same way but also requires special measures and the accommodation of differences," for women, people with disabilities, visible minorities, and Indigenous peoples.

The next time you walk into a shoe store, take note that not every person is sold the identical shoe. "One size fits all" may sound like Charter compliance, but it overlooks the undeniable fact that we are not all the same, our differences need to be accommodated; and equality

In Search of Dignity. Harvey Max Chochinov, Oxford University Press. © Oxford University Press 2025.
DOI: 10.1093/9780197805145.003.0029

means exiting the store with an equal likelihood that our feet are comfortable.

For Canadians, being equal under and before the law means having equal opportunities to flourish and thrive. Deluding ourselves that providing MAiD for mental illness is somehow in the service of equality or the avoidance of discrimination and exceptionalism, is responding to an empty hollow soundbite, shouted by MAiD proponents who have lost sight of what it will take to help the mentally ill flourish and thrive, which is access to treatment and support.

Protecting, Caring for the Mentally Ill by Harvey Max Chochinov. An earlier version of this essay first appeared in *Winnipeg Free Press* on March 22nd, 2016.

Who but those who have experienced it can appreciate the soul-crushing anguish of mental illness? Afflictions of the mind can be paralyzing and fundamentally change the way we perceive ourselves (I am worthless), anticipate the future (my prospects are hopeless) and experience the world (life is unfair and unforgiving). The combination of self-loathing, hopelessness and despair can tragically lead to suicide.

Parliament's joint committee on physician-assisted death, nevertheless, urged the federal government not to exclude individuals with psychiatric conditions from being considered eligible. Their reasoning comes down to this: mental suffering is no less profound than physical suffering, so denying individuals with mental illness access to physician-hastened death would be discriminatory and a violation of their Charter rights.

People with mental illness are no strangers to discrimination. Two-thirds suffer in silence for fear of rejection and mistreatment. Only one in five children who need mental health services receive them, either because of concerns they will be stigmatized or supports are simply not available. Doors are constantly being closed on the mentally ill, denying them stable employment, social opportunities, secure food and housing, and sometimes fundamental protections under our criminal justice system. They are marginalized, victimized and vilified. Mental illness is one of the best predictors, more so than poverty, of inequitable access to health care in Canada. People with severe mental illness die about 25 years earlier than adults in the general population.

Making a fairness argument for the availability of physician-hastened death for a group of people treated so unfairly seems a cruel irony. In Oregon, having a psychiatric condition does not preclude eligibility for physician-assisted suicide. However, that condition must not impair the patient's capacity to give consent and must, as in every other eligible case, occur alongside a medical condition with a prognosis of less than six months. Experts I met who are involved in Oregon's Death With Dignity Act, in place 17 years now, could not fathom the idea of providing assisted suicide purely based on non-terminal psychiatric disorders.

In the Netherlands, Belgium and Luxembourg, psychological suffering stemming from either a physical or emotional condition is considered a valid legal basis for physician-hastened death. They account for a small but growing minority of death-hastening cases. Last month, a critically important study was published in the journal *JAMA Psychiatry* by American psychiatrist Scott Kim. Kim and his team reviewed 66 case summaries, published online by the Dutch regional euthanasia review committee between 2011 and 2014, of people who had received either euthanasia or assisted suicide for psychiatric reasons. The majority were women, with issues including depression, psychosis, post-traumatic stress disorder, anxiety, substance abuse, various forms of cognitive impairment (intellectual disability, early dementia), eating disorders, prolonged grief and autism. Most had personality disorders and were described as socially isolated and lonely. In one quarter of instances, despite differences of opinion between physicians, death hastening proceeded. In about one third of cases initially refused, most were carried out by new physicians willing to comply.

The parliamentary committee's position seems premised on the recognition physical suffering and mental suffering can be equally devastating. That does not mean, however, they can be approached the same. The nature of mental illness often leads people to see themselves as worthless, to believe their situation is hopeless, and to perceive—often reflected through society's judgmental gaze—that their lives have little value. But this context should help us see a death-hastening response is fraught with hazard and runs counter to a recovery-oriented practice advocated by the Mental Health Commission of Canada.

Like all Canadians, people with mental illness have rights that are protected under the Constitution. And like all Canadians, these rights need to be balanced against the interests of a free and just society, wherein vulnerable persons must be protected. The most effective protections health care providers offer patients are built on the foundation of a caring and committed therapeutic relationship. For patients whose illness tends toward self-destruction, and for patients whose suffering is rooted in social conditions such as loneliness, a physician-assisted death option will crack that relational foundation. Current evidence indicates vulnerable persons will fall through that crack.

The committee, in its wisdom, expressed confidence physicians would be able to figure this out. Hopefully, as lawmakers draft legislation in the days ahead, deeper wisdom will prevail.

30

Intensive, Compassionate Caring—Not Medical Assistance in Dying—Is Most Effective Way to Address Mental Illness

Few Canadians likely recall the Senate of Canada introducing an amendment to Bill-C7, which would have allowed mental illness as the sole underlying medical condition to be eligible for medical assistance in dying (MAiD). This was to come into effect in March 2023 but was delayed to March 2024, and further delayed until March 2027. Backers of the amendment told the Special Parliamentary Committee on MAiD that mentally ill patients have historically been stigmatized, marginalized, victimized, and discriminated against. We also know they often live in poverty and lack food and housing security and opportunities most of us take for granted; they also struggle to access mental health services, which are in desperately short supply. And yet, without addressing any of these injustices, proponents argued that withholding the option of MAiD would be egregious and discriminatory. It seems disingenuous that for people whose lives have been distorted by inequities and lack of support, treatment, and security, the battleground chosen to protect their Charter right to equal treatment under the law is MAiD.

MAiD proponents told the Parliamentary Committee that MAiD is not the same as suicide and the two can be distinguished. Despite that, the Canadian Association of Suicide Prevention said, "By the very definition of suicide, which is the act of killing oneself, if the condition from which they are suffering is not killing them, then the act of providing medical assistance in dying is doctor-assisted suicide." At one point during an appearance on CBC's Fifth Estate, David Lammetti, then the Justice Minister, described MAiD as "a species of suicide."

Proponents have tried to assure parliamentarians they should have great faith in MAiD assessors trained to perform these evaluations and sort through these issues. They were reminded that a national MAiD

In Search of Dignity. Harvey Max Chochinov, Oxford University Press. © Oxford University Press 2025.
DOI: 10.1093/9780197805145.003.0030

training program is well underway, with the Canadian Association of MAiD Assessors and Practitioners (CAMAP) receiving $3.3 million in funding from Health Canada to develop and implement a national curriculum aiming to provide high-quality MAiD training to healthcare practitioners across Canada. Journalist Alex Raikin reported in the New Atlantis *that CAMAP "has sat on credible evidence by its own members that people are being driven to euthanasia by credit card debt, poor housing, and difficulties getting medical care." Raikin also documented that MAiD trainees are being taught that when socioeconomic reasons are driving MAiD, if they themselves feel disinclined to provide it, "you'll then have to refer the person on to somebody else, who may hopefully fulfill the request in the end." An instructor was recorded telling MAiD trainees that "you can ask as many clinicians as you want or need" to get the opinion you are after. "Disagreement doesn't mean you must stop," MAiD instructor Ellen Wiebe[a] told trainees. "It is rare for assessors to have patients who have unmet needs, but it does happen. Usually, these unmet needs are around loneliness and poverty. As all Canadians have rights to an assisted death, people who are lonely or poor also have those rights."*

When the Special Joint Committee on Medical Assistance in Dying submitted its report, they concluded Canada is not ready to expand MAiD for mental illness. The government then recommended a delay until March 2027. The dissenting report admonished the committee for not filling its mandate and suggested their majority report should not be accepted by the Government of Canada. One member of the Joint Committee, Senator Stanley Kutcher, said, "There's historical precedents in the Senate for addressing some of these issues [differently] than the House addresses them" and that the Senate must "protect against the tyranny of the majority."

It is worth recalling the Supreme Court decision in Carter vs. Canada, *in which it stated that the invalidation of s. 241(b) and s. 14 of the Criminal Code was "intended to respond to the factual circumstances in this case"— that is, the factual circumstances that were the focus of the Court's analysis were those of Gloria Taylor, who suffered from amyotrophic lateral sclerosis (ALS), a fatal neurodegenerative disease. The Court stated it was making "no pronouncement on other situations where physician-assisted dying may be sought," noting that assistance in dying in other situations, such as for*

---

[a] Wiebe testified before a parliamentary committee in 2023 that she had assessed about 750 people, of whom she provided MAiD to 430.

*"minors or persons with psychiatric disorders or minor medical conditions"
would not fall within the parameters suggested in its reasons. Clearly, they
were unfamiliar with the nature of helium (see Chapter 27).*

**Intensive, Compassionate Caring—Not Medical Assistance in Dying—Is
Most Effective Way to Address Mental Illness** by Harvey Max Chochinov.
An earlier version of this essay first appeared in *Toronto Star* on December
30th, 2023.

It's time to put the brakes on Medical Assistance in Dying (MAiD) in Canada
for those whose sole underlying medical condition is mental illness.

The federal government has tasked the Special Joint Committee on
Medical Assistance in Dying to determine if Canada is ready to extend MAiD
eligibility, starting in March 2024, to patients with mental illness alone.
Despite those convinced it is time, and safe, to launch what amounts to "psychiatric euthanasia," the Special Committee must pay attention to a murmur
of protest that has grown to a roar: "Ottawa, we've got a problem."

There are two main reasons to abort this mission. Current MAiD eligibility requires a person have a grievous and irremediable medical condition.
Unlike some cancers, and many neurodegenerative disorders, no mental
disorder can be described as irremediable. To be sure, there are individuals
whose mental affliction won't improve, despite myriad treatments or psychosocial interventions. But there is currently no way to predict which patients
won't get better.

Studies of prognostic accuracy show psychiatrists are wrong half the time.[1]
I have cared for patients struggling with chronic suicidality; patients I worried might one day take their lives. I recall a woman with mind-numbing
depression, who teetered precariously between life and death. One day, after
years of countless drug trials, hospitalizations, electroconvulsive therapy,
and various psychosocial interventions, she arrived for her appointment—
three weeks into starting a new antidepressant—with a grin on her face.

"The door is purple," she declared. I told her the door had always been
purple, to which she replied, "I know, but now I care."

Before that moment, no one—not me, not her friends or family and not
anyone on The Special Joint Committee on Medical Assistance in Dying,
nor any MAiD assessor—could have predicted her recovery.

Intensive, unwavering, compassionate care and caring—not MAiD—offers the most effective way to address this kind of suffering.

The other reason not to launch psychiatric euthanasia is our inability to determine suicidality from those requesting MAiD whose sole underlying medical condition is mental illness. According to the Canadian Association for Suicide Prevention, someone not dying because of their condition, such as a mental disorder alone, seeking death is, by definition, suicidal.[2]

Similarly, the first item listed by the American Association of Suicidology differentiating physician hastened death and suicide is the patient must be dying. That certainly does not characterize patients who are mentally ill.

Despite this, the Special Joint Committee is being told by some MAiD expansionists, "suicidality and having a reason to want to die are not at all the same." We can say "six" and "half-dozen" are not the same as many times as we like. If we repeat it frequently, consistently and without equivocation, it might even sound convincing, but that doesn't make it true.

Patients struggling with suicidality often have a reason to want to die, based on, for example, self-loathing, feeling a burden or becoming worn down pursuing care and support that could sustain them. In those instances, the line between MAiD and suicide simply vanishes.

Most proponents of psychiatric euthanasia are prepared to overlook all of this, claiming failure to expand MAiD to the mentally ill is discriminatory. Avoiding discrimination does not mean everyone is treated the same, but rather, that everyone gets equal access to what they need to thrive.

Claiming a lethal injection for mentally ill patients is a respectful, compassionate, and necessary response to their suffering is akin to arguing the virtue of helping people to the balcony of a burning building so they might choose death, rather than sorting out how to control or extinguish the fire.

Time and again, committee members have asked witnesses when Canada's psychiatric euthanasia program can be launched. I would suggest they behave like NASA. When a potentially catastrophic problem is identified before blast-off, space engineers don't set an arbitrary new launch date, no more so than Health Canada announces a random release date of a new drug discovered to have unacceptable side-effects.

Members of the Special Joint Committee must listen and exercise reason, wisdom, and restraint in the face of fierce opposition.

"Ottawa, we have a problem." The federal government would be well advised to scrap this mission. But if it insists on moving forward, launch should proceed only when the problems are solved, and not a moment sooner.

References

1. Nicolini ME, Jardas E, Zarate CA, et al. Irremediability in psychiatric euthanasia: examining the objective standard. *Psychol Med*. 2023;53(12):5729–5747.
2. Canadian Association of Suicide Prevention. CASP issues statement about MAiD for mental illness. https://suicideprevention.ca/media/casp-issues-statement-about-maid-for-mental-illness/ (last accessed December 23, 2024).

31

Is Medical Assistance in Dying Part of Palliative Care?

My friend's wife spent her last 2 weeks of life on an inpatient palliative care ward. While experiencing cancer-related pain, she was told that medical assistance in dying (MAiD) was something she might want to consider. To the very end she needed reassurance that medications weren't being used to hasten her death.

This vignette was meant to preface the article reprinted in this chapter, "Is Medical Assistance in Dying Part of Palliative Medicine?" While it didn't appear in the final publication, it was nevertheless the inspiration for writing this piece.

There is clearly something about MAiD that distinguishes it from the rest of medicine. While some argue it is just another treatment option, as was the case with my friend's wife, it can undermine expectations that those providing care will do nothing to hasten death. And can a prescription for death be considered treatment or, more broadly, part of medicine? When I chaired the federal government's External Panel on Options for a Legislative Response to Carter vs. Canada, I had the opportunity to ask those questions of individuals deeply engaged in death-hastening practices. While in Holland, I spoke with a leading euthanasia proponent who told me he didn't consider death hastening a medical act, but rather "a societal act." In other words, he saw this as a social policy issue, supported by political decisions to make euthanasia and assisted suicide available to Dutch citizens.

Our panel also visited Oregon, where we met people who provide services available under that state's Death with Dignity Act. I asked one physician whose practice included assisted suicide if he considered this part of medicine. His response was unequivocal: "I do not consider it a medical act," he said, "but I do consider it an act of love." This suggested to me that whatever our understanding of MAiD, it is unlike the rest of medicine. (Some ideas

In Search of Dignity. Harvey Max Chochinov, Oxford University Press. © Oxford University Press 2025.
DOI: 10.1093/9780197805145.003.0031

have a long gestation period, given the article below was written 8 years after our panel submitted its final report.[a]*)*

MAiD is an end-of-life option (although this is no longer accurate in the wake of Bill C7 [see Chapter 27*]) as well as a life-ending option. Like other near-death transactions, such as consulting a lawyer, meeting with an estate planner, or speaking with a funeral director, it is possible for assisted dying to be a coordinated service, albeit organized and administered outside the house of medicine. Suffering patients require knowledgeable, evidence-based care, centered on hope, commitment, and affirmation. Embodying that approach, while arbitrating the option of a lethal injection or lethal overdose, is like trying to inhale and exhale simultaneously: It simply isn't possible.*

Is Medical Assistance in Dying Part of Palliative Care? Harvey Max Chochinov and Joseph J. Fins. *JAMA*. 2024;332(14):1137–1138. Reproduced with permission of the American Medical Association.

Whatever one's view on medical assistance in dying (MAID), an underlying question is whether it should be considered part of palliative care. The Canadian Hospice Palliative Care Association takes the stance that MAID "definitionally fall[s] outside of the scope of palliative care."[1] This is a historical perspective dating to Hippocratic injunctions against a fatal draught. But with the advent of euthanasia and assisted suicide as legal life ending options in various jurisdictions, the insistence on separation between palliative care and MAID has been questioned. Although some assert the purposeful hastening of death should always be outside the scope of medical practice,[2] others contend that respect for patient choice at life's end is central to modern notions of patient-centered care. Setting those considerations aside, this article seeks to determine whether MAID is part of palliative care, based on characteristics embedded within the practice of medicine.

Palliative Care, MAID, and Medicine

Although the place of MAID within palliative care remains contentious, there is universal agreement that palliative care is part of medicine. Hence,

---

[a] Consultations on Physician-Assisted Dying: Summary of Results and Key Findings, December 15, 2015. https://www.justice.gc.ca/eng/rp-pr/other-autre/pad-amm/toc-tdm.html

MAID can only be considered part of palliative care if this practice resides within the house of medicine. If medicine does not include it, neither can palliative care.

Determining whether MAID is a medical treatment is worth considering through a useful heuristic offered by Thomas et al,[3] which describes canons of therapy. The first of these canons, restoration, "counsels that the goal of all treatment is to restore the patient, as much as possible, to homeostatic equilibrium." Restoration aims to return the patient to a previously held state of wellness, capacity, or disposition. In advancing terminal illness, this means redefining homeostatic equilibrium by pursuing comfort care, the amelioration of pain, and to the extent possible, returning the patient to a state of greater engagement with their friends and family. These activities are the mainstay of palliative care. It is hard to conceive of MAID as restorative because the very act makes any return impossible.

The next canon is means-end proportionality, which "holds that every treatment should be well-fitted to the intended goal or end." One can only judge the proportionality of the means as it relates to the ends, which in palliative care is the relief of suffering. It is difficult to regard death as "well-fitted" because nonexistence negates alternative means to address pain. Death cannot be titrated and trialed; hence, it does not qualify as a therapeutic, which means its pursuit resides outside the realm of medicine.

The next canon is parsimony, "which maintains that only as much therapeutic force as is necessary should be used to achieve the therapeutic goal." This is a central feature of good medical practice, whether it be in the choice of antibiotics or a surgical intervention. This tailoring of a therapy to a specific condition, drawing on evidence-based guidelines, is violated under MAID, where patient preference effectively dictates practice. By way of example, Canadians seeking MAID are under no obligation to try other treatments they deem unacceptable. In those instances, physicians may have to dispense with parsimony—despite their clinical judgment pointing toward other options—yielding to the patient's intent on receiving MAID.

The final canon, discretion, is closely related to parsimony and scope of practice. Discretion "counsels that an awareness of the limits of medical knowledge and practice should guide all treatment decisions." Since MAID was launched in Canada, eligibility has broadened from those whose deaths are reasonably foreseeable, to individuals who are not dying but living with disability; with consideration now being given to mental illness, children, and those anticipating the loss of mental capacity. Although some may see this as affirming individual autonomy, ethicist Paul Ramsey[4] reminds us that physicians must recognize that the function of medicine is not to relieve the human condition of the human condition.

MAID and the Patient-Physician Relationship

In 2015, the British Medical Association's end-of-life care and physician-assisted dying project examined perceptions and experiences of end-of-life care and palliative care.[5] Some members of the public indicated legalizing death hastening would enhance their physicians' ability to provide them a good death and more choice. In contrast, others said it would undermine trust and increase their fear of physicians, particularly for individuals who are elderly, disabled, vulnerable, or religious; individuals who are opposed to MAID; and individuals who see themselves as a burden. Although some physicians felt it could help them provide a good death, accommodate patient preferences, and improve end-of-life communication, others cautioned it might increase fear and suspicion of physicians (including hospices and palliative care physicians), harm their reputation, and change their fundamental role as healers.

MAID undermines the patient-physician relationship by violating the principle of non-abandonment, even when it is well intended. At the height of patients' distress, MAID truncates care and eliminates the possibility of healing. This distinguishes it from palliative medicine, which embraces patient and family at life's end with fidelity and relationality extending into bereavement care for survivors.

MAID, Hope, and Palliative Care

Unlike MAID, palliative care embodies an evidence-based response to human suffering. Intensive caring[6] assures patients that they won't be abandoned; affirms their worth and ongoing value; takes an interest in them as people; sustains hope for possibilities of finding meaning and purpose; and maintains therapeutic humility when problems are intractable. It is impossible to sustain this therapeutic stance when assessing a patient's readiness for MAID. The former entails holistic medical care, whereas the latter shifts to a legalistic paradigm centered on determining eligibility for MAID.

Practitioner Ambivalence and Policy Considerations

The moral argument—that the taking of human life is wrong—does not appear to be the most dominant ideological fence separating palliative care from MAID. Although some argue that MAID is bad for society and antithetical to the role of being a health care professional,[2] others contend it provides those who are suffering an autonomous choice to end their lives. The policy arguments separating MAID and palliative care are rooted in the notion that palliative care affirms life, regards dying as a normal process, and is committed to "neither hasten nor postpone death."[1] Organizations representing palliative care have been resolute in asserting that MAID falls beyond their mandate. That said, the American Academy of Hospice and Palliative Medicine[7] characterizes its position as "studied neutrality," which we take as emblematic of its ambivalence.

This ambivalence also permeates variable responses in different states and nations. A recent international scoping review examined the relation between palliative care and assisted dying where lawful.[8] Notwithstanding differences across constituencies, it describes the relationship between palliative care and MAID as varied and sometimes combined, including supportive, neutral, coexisting, not mutually exclusive, integrated, synergistic, cooperative, collaborative, opposed, ambivalent, and conflicted. The 2 included Swiss studies indicated that physicians do not actively participate in offering assisted suicide as part of palliative care and do not consider it a medical act. The single Canadian study of physicians reported that some agreed to take part in all aspects of MAID, others to undertake MAID assessments but do not administer the lethal medications, whereas others would not agree to take part in any aspect of MAID.[9] In Belgium, where the relationship is described as highly integrated, the review cites a lack of detail and nuanced insight regarding "how euthanasia is introduced within a palliative care context and whether and how this varies within and across institutions or professional groups."[8] The authors concluded that "none of the selected articles explain how the synergistic relationship takes form in practice," raising the question of how to provide patient-centered multidisciplinary palliative care for patients interested in opting for an assisted death.[4]

These data suggest that medicine is uncomfortable with MAID because it resides outside conventional practice.[10] Administering a lethal medication does not make it a medical act, albeit health care professional involvement and a medical environment provide an air of credibility and legitimacy.

Considering MAID as a legal intervention and a rights issue, centered on a singular intervention of ending life, reveals the complexity of an act currently cloaked as medical care. Although this may cause patients and practitioners to feel less sanguine toward MAID, some health care professionals will continue to offer this service, albeit outside the scope of medicine. This shift in perspective may also garner additional resources to promote care and deepen understanding for patients who are suffering or nearing death.

References

1. Canadian Hospice Palliative Care Association. CHPCA's position statement on MAiD—2023 update. https://www.chpca.ca/wp-content/uploads/2024/07/CHPCAs-Position-Statement-on-MAiD-%E2%80%93-2023-Update.pdf (accessed July 20, 2024).
2. Fins JJ, Morrissey MB. Reflections on "aid in dying" and the paradox of "achieving death": avoiding the confluence of language and ideology at life's end. *Health Law J.* 2018;23:59–65.
3. Thomas C, Alici Y, Breitbart W, Bruera E, Blackler. Accessed March 1, 2024. https://www.bma.org.uk/media/4399/bma-doctor-patient-relationship-and-pad-aug-2021.pdf
4. Ramsey P. The Patient as Person. Yale University Press; 1970.
5. British Medical Association. Physician-assisted-dying: the doctor patient relationship. August 2021. Accessed March 1, 2024. https://www.bma.org.uk/media/4399/bma-doctor-patient-relationshipand-pad-aug-2021.pdf
6. Chochinov HM. Intensive caring: reminding patients they matter. *J Clin Oncol.* 2023;41(16):2884–2887. doi:10.1200/JCO.23.00042
7. American Academy of Hospice and Palliative Medicine. Statement on physician assisted death. June 24, 2016. https://aahpm.org/positions/pad (accessed May 24, 2024).
8. Gerson SM, Koksvik GH, Richards N, et al. The relationship of palliative care with assisted dying where assisted dying is lawful: a systematic scoping review of the literature. *J Pain Symptom Manage.* 2020;59(6):1287–1303.
9. Wales J, Isenberg SR, Wegier P, et al. Providing medical assistance in dying within a home palliative care program in Toronto, Canada: an observational study of the first year of experience. *J Palliat Med.* 2018;21(11):1573–1579.
10. Preston N, Payne S, Ost S. Breaching the stalemate on assisted dying: it's time to move beyond a medicalised approach. *BMJ.* 2023;382:1968.

SECTION 5
PERSONAL REFLECTIONS

32

Cruising for a Bruising

For 20 years I've gotten away with it. His lawyers have never contacted my lawyers, and for that I'm eternally grateful. Comparing resources, it's a case of Knight versus Day. But is reprinting this piece tempting fate, and could keeping this from coming to his attention be Mission: Impossible—The Final Reckoning? I mean really, what are the chances that someone knows someone, who knows someone, who arranges a tell-all Interview with the Vampire. His American-made litigation would see me lose my shirt, lose my home, and end up looking for low-cost housing in the Space Station, with a message from Jack Reacher saying "Never Go Back." Despite all I've tried to achieve in this life, it would all come to Oblivion.

Cruising for a Bruising. Harvey M. Chochinov. Cruising for a bruising. *Palliative & Supportive Care*, 2005;3(3):171. Reproduced with permission of Cambridge University Press.

Perhaps I best not mention his name; his lawyers, after all, are much more familiar with The Color of Money than mine will ever be. Nevertheless, these outrageous rantings by one of Hollywood's alleged Top Guns—denouncing psychiatry and challenging the legitimacy of psychiatric illness—has got to stop.

Claiming he has a Firm grip on the facts, he defends an ideology that refers to psychiatry as a "Nazi Science"; one can only imagine how Holocaust survivor and psychoanalyst, Victor Frankl—author of "Man's Search for Meaning"—might have responded to such a vile claim. He further describes psychiatry as a pseudoscience; that the key to beating depression, attention deficit disorder, and psychotic disorders is not some evil drug Cocktail, but rather proper exercise, ample vitamins, and plain good living.

Now, I wasn't Born on the 4th of July, or yesterday for that matter, but surely, the ability to play the role of an authority does not confer authority status or authority

In Search of Dignity. Harvey Max Chochinov, Oxford University Press. © Oxford University Press 2025.
DOI: 10.1093/9780197805145.003.0032

knowledge. Conflating one with the other is Risky Business, with the potential for much Collateral damage. For example, 154,000 people apparently wrote their thanks for his public diatribe; he did not, however, disclose how many bothered to register their objections. Let us imagine that each of those correspondents was someone with a chronic major mental illness. According to his prescription, All the Right Moves would include stopping medication, abandoning psychiatric support, popping vitamins, and perhaps taking up an exercise class.

Now I don't mean to Rain, Man, on your parade, but do you understand the despair of profound, soul crushing depression, the anguish of feeling one's mind spinning out of control, or the terror of entering into a mental space well past Losin' It?

The judicious use of psychopharmaceuticals, as part of comprehensive psychiatric care, can make the difference between life and death, and while this may not jive with your picture of "the ideal scene for life," whoever said life was ideal—except perhaps in the movies.

Over the past few decades, more than a Few Good Men and women have amassed evidence, within the fields of epidemiology, psychiatry, psychology, neurochemistry, pharmacology, neuroimaging, and genetics, establishing the validity of various psychiatric disorders. As you correctly point out, there is no simple "blood test" to confirm these diagnoses, but the same could be said of many medical conditions. Pain, for example, cannot be diagnosed on the basis of a blood test, and yet clearly exists.

In my field of end-of-life care, the skillful application of analgesic medication, along with comprehensive palliative care well before the time to play Taps can make all the difference between anguish and good quality of life.

So why bother embarking on this Mission: Impossible, by taking issue with this Young Gun? It is because most of us will forever remain Outsiders to the experience of being a mega-celebrity. This rarified status confers power and influence, including the Endless Love and adoration of fans and followers worldwide.

The likes of Bono, Geldof, and Jolie are using their celebrity to try and reshape the world into a place that is Far and Away from a planet plagued by poverty, pandemics, and strife.

So why squander the opportunity of your celebrity? Worse yet, why use it to do a disservice to people whose suffering renders them so vulnerable? I know, I know, you have read the history of psychiatry, and you have reviewed the literature. But alas, you must have done so with your Eyes Wide Shut.

33

Reflections on Losing a Friend

It's hard to believe Marcy Dempsey died more than 22 years ago. As I predicted in a piece I published shortly after her death, she has not been forgotten. My friendship with her husband, Neil, remains steadfast. I have watched him raise their three wonderful daughters and celebrate the arrival of three grandchildren. Twenty-two years. The world stands still for no one.

A few months before dying of metastatic breast cancer, Marcy and I had a phone call that is etched in my memory. I'd been selected to receive an award that would draw significant public attention, and Marcy wanted to know how I was feeling about it. I told her about my discomfort, borne out of a sense that others were as deserving and my unhealthy imposter syndrome. Marcy was smart and emotionally intelligent. She knew how to listen and how to deftly unravel myriad psychological and spiritual threads. While I can't recount her exact words, her response hit me like a lightning bolt. She asked me if I planned to attend the event, which I did. That being the case, she said I had two choices: to be fully present and take in the moment or allow distraction and self-doubt to make me a no-show.

Whether it was the message, the messenger, or both, the effect was immediate, truly a moment of epiphany. Marcy's lesson was to show up for life and to be mindful and take it in, fully and thoughtfully. We can't always control what life dishes out, but we can choose how to respond. For more than two decades I've held her words and wisdom close to my heart.

I don't know if Marcy understood her power. I hope she knew that her indominable spirit influenced everyone whose life she touched. Over the years I've come to appreciate the importance of knowing one's power. Each one of us has distinctive qualities, gifts, and perspectives. Embracing your power—knowing that never before nor ever again will there be one exactly like you (see Chapter 37*)—allows you to shape the world in unique ways. For instance, I have occasionally been asked to officiate Canadian citizenship ceremonies. This involves swearing in people who have come to this country from around the world, representing all walks of life. As the officiant, I am seen to have certain qualities and status, power if you will*

In Search of Dignity. Harvey Max Chochinov, Oxford University Press. © Oxford University Press 2025.
DOI: 10.1093/9780197805145.003.0033

(the fact that I don't think of myself in those terms is not the point here).
Embracing that power can move people and leave an indelible mark on the
day they swear allegiance to King and Country. Which is why I tell them: "I
leave you now with my warmest wishes for a long, peaceful, and prosperous
life in this, your chosen land. Canada is a great country, not despite you
being a part of us, but because you are a part of us. I am proud to call each of
you fellow citizens!"

Granted they are only words, but I can tell by the look on the face of every
new citizen taking their oath that those words move and resonate deeply.

Knowing your power as a healthcare provider is important. Don't
squander it, don't dismiss it, don't underestimate its potency, and don't
be seduced by it. Tell patients you care about them; that you value them;
that you are committed to looking after them; and that you won't abandon
them, no matter what. Those words and sentiments are powerful and will
resonate deeply with people who see you as embodying the role of healer.
I think Marcy would have understood this. Decades later, I think I do too.

Reflections on Losing a Friend. Harvey Max Chochinov, Reflections
on losing a friend. *Palliative & Supportive Care*, 2003;1(2):109–109.
Reproduced with permission of Cambridge University Press .

Four days after Mother's Day, May 15, 2003, my dear friend Marcy Dempsey
passed away. Her personal reflection, "A Toolbox for Living: Cancer
Reflections," can be read within the current issue of *Palliative and Supportive
Care*. I do wish she were still here, not so much just to see this piece come
out, but to grace us longer with her gentle spirit, boundless energy, and sage
wisdom.

It feels odd to begin this, my first contribution to P&SC, on such a personal, intimate note. But then again, this journal was launched with the
intent of taking its readership to places not frequently found in other
publications. With a mandate to address the psychosocial, spiritual, and existential dimensions of end-of-life care, P&SC will need to include content
that speaks to the profoundly personal and fundamentally human aspects
of end-of-life care. This will take on various conventional forms, including
clinical trial reports, literature reviews, and an assortment of scholarly papers. However, probing the meaning and impact of life-altering losses and

expanding the field of inquiry around end-of-life care will require an open-ness to various forms of expression. In that regard, personal reflections such as Marcy's have so very much to teach us.

Marcy was diagnosed with breast cancer five years ago and died just shy of her 40th birthday. Throughout her illness, her vigorous commitment to being a mother, wife, friend, and life-long learner was unwavering. Like so many people living with a life-limiting condition, Marcy was looking for answers and, ultimately as it turned out, for tangible meaning. She would occasionally ask me for book recommendations and always seemed touched and enlightened by these literary retreats; once, feeling the pressure of wanting to keep up my track record, I asked her what sort of book she was up for next. She replied, "something that will give me insights." To the very end, she was trying to figure things out and trying to make sense of what was happening to her.

While she clearly tried to prepare herself for death, at the same time, she fully immersed herself in the joy and challenges of living. Perhaps this is a variation on what Avery Weisman referred to as "middle knowledge"; the ability to anticipate death, while simultaneously planning on life. Recent studies have focused on the importance of meaning and purpose as funda-mental components of quality life among patients who are terminally ill. That being the case, one of the great challenges facing palliative care practitioners is how to identify these sources of meaning and use them to engender hope and purpose toward the end of life. Whether the language we use falls within the realm of psychological, spiritual, or existential discourse, these are com-pelling issues that demand our attention. "A Toolbox for Living" is one re-markable woman's personal journey through this landscape of meaning and purpose, as her life draws to a close. Marcy died surrounded by a circle of friends, who softly chanted her favorite Hebrew melodies as she passed from this world into the next. As for her fear of being forgotten, I am convinced that she helped fill each of our "toolboxes for living" with gifts that will last a lifetime.

34

Barney's Version

Observations from the Edge

I'm often asked about the "right thing" to say or do when someone is facing serious illness or nearing death (see Chapter 17*). There are many wrong turns one can take, like giving false reassurances, pretending nothing bad is happening, or rationalizing that things are less dire than they really are or that this is part of some larger cosmic plan. These unhelpful platitudes usually reflect a sense of helplessness and a desperate attempt to make the person, and ourselves, feel better.*

Understanding Intensive Caring (see Chapter 19*) provides a way to let go of expectations to fix what can't be fixed and includes concepts of Therapeutic Presence and Therapeutic Humility, which are fundamental tools when entering this exquisitely delicate space. Setting aside what one says, it is important to know that showing up and listening convey caring and affirmation: "Who you are, what you have to say, the memories or wisdom you choose to share, those things still matter. You still matter." Listening and being attentive and interested are critical therapeutic currency.*

It is also important to understand certain aspects of this emotional landscape, starting with the developmental psychologist Erik Erikson. Erikson outlined key tasks people face at different points in their psychosocial development. Each stage contains a conflict between two opposing states that shape personality.[a] Successful completion of each stage sees the acquisition of certain virtues, which can be used in facing subsequent crises. The latter stages in Erikson's schema include generativity versus stagnation and, toward the end of life, integrity versus despair.

While the notion of generativity was influential in the conception and development of Dignity Therapy, it also applies to understanding what matters to people entering middle age and beyond. Generativity is about feeling one

---

[a] McLeod S. Erik Erikson's stages of psychosocial development. Simply Psychology. https://www.simplypsychology.org/erik-erikson.html, updated January 25, 2024.

In Search of Dignity. Harvey Max Chochinov, Oxford University Press. © Oxford University Press 2025.
DOI: 10.1093/9780197805145.003.0034

has made a difference in some personal, meaningful way. It often involves concern for others and a desire to contribute to those we will leave behind, for instance through parenting, being a role model or a leader, or doing good deeds, good work, or creative output the individual deems valuable. Lack of generativity results in stagnation, which means feeling unproductive, uninvolved, and self-absorbed, lacking a sense of growth, and feeling empty. While Dame Cicely Saunders famously said, "You matter because you are you," the nature of generativity points to those things that really matter to each person.

Erikson's final stage of psychosocial development is integrity versus despair, which begins at approximately age 65 and ends at death. This is a time of contemplation and reflection, with those who can find a sense of fulfillment and meaning experiencing ego integrity. Having a sense of closure and completeness fosters acceptance of death and mitigates fear of dying. On the other hand, those who feel regret and disappointment in life may experience despair, bitterness, depression, hopelessness, and a fear of death.

I believe Erikson's notion of integrity includes the task of integration. This is the only time one can contemplate the puzzle of life with all the pieces on the table. Erikson described this as an attempt to put life into perspective to find personal meaning. In the 1960s Dr. Robert Butler, a psychiatrist who specialized in working with the geriatric population, introduced what he referred to as Reminiscence Therapy. He recognized that as people reach their later years, reminiscence offers a way for them to connect with their past and evaluate their lives. He called this concept "life review", which I believe offers another way of putting the pieces together.

This article is about my good friend and colleague, Barney, and the final conversation we had before he died of pancreatic cancer. I'm not surprised we found ourselves talking about his interest in military history, medical aid in dying, and contemplating the nature of death. It was by no means our first time doing so. While cancer found him stuck in his bed, our conversation placed him exactly where he always enjoyed being, which was intellectually on the edge of his seat. And it is no coincidence that with death approaching, Barney found himself sharing special memories of his life, perhaps in some way contemplating how all the pieces fit.

The next time you anticipate sharing time with someone nearing death and wonder what to say or what to talk about, think about the importance of listening, think about Erik Erikson, think about Robert Butler—and think about Barney.

Barney's Version Observations from the Edge. Harvey M. Chochinov. *Palliative & Supportive Care*, 2006;4(3):217–218. Reproduced with permission from Cambridge University Press.

My good friend and colleague Barney Sneiderman died yesterday. A few months ago he was diagnosed with pancreatic cancer; the day before yesterday, after failed trials of chemotherapy and staying at home—with community palliative care supports—as long as possible, he determined it was time to enter one of our city's inpatient palliative care units. Less than a day later, he was gone. Some readers of *Palliative & Supportive Care* may be familiar with Barney, through his various published works. As a professor of law at the University of Manitoba, he was known for his expertise in health issues and the law and biomedical ethics. He was a frequent speaker to medical professionals on medicolegal subjects, and had a cross-appointment with the Faculty of Medicine at the University of Manitoba. Besides his many publications, the book he coauthored, *Canadian Medical Law: An Introduction for Physicians, Nurses and Other Health Care Professionals*, third edition, is considered an authoritative work on legal issues relating to patient care and treatment and addresses the most frequent and pressing concerns facing health care professionals and the lawyers who advise them.

I cannot say that I have ever known anyone quite like Barney. He was an interesting combination of kindness, intellectual intensity, and nervous energy. In fact, to coin a phrase that aptly applies, Barney had what I would call "intellectual akathesia"[1]; the inability to ever set one's mind entirely at rest. An illustrative case example might offer some clarity. About 15 years ago, Barney and his wife Carla were in Hawaii, together with their then very young children. My own family happened to be vacationing in Hawaii at the time. One afternoon, along with other friends, we all had the good fortune of spending some very memorable time together. It was one of those glorious idyllic days, when the intense Hawaiian sun, the turquoise blue water, and the fragrantly scented air made you feel that in all creation, nothing could compare. Barney and I were walking along the water's edge, having fallen somewhat behind the rest of the group.

Finding ourselves alone, Barney immediately began talking about one of his favorite topics, physician-assisted suicide. While I did my best to politely disengage from this soliloquy, he went on citing case law, legal precedents, and the like. Finally, no longer being able to tolerate this one-sided conversation, I said, "Barney, we're in paradise. I DON'T WANT to be talking about physician-assisted suicide!!" We strolled onward, while I briefly considered whether I had been somewhat harsh in achieving this glorious silence. Not more than a few seconds later Barney turned to me and said—completely straight-faced and unfazed—"Well, I'm really interested in the Holocaust."

Barney spent a great deal of his professional life thinking, speaking, and writing about death. In fact, during our final conversation, which took place midafternoon the day before he died, he told me how pleased he was that his final publication placed our names side by side (companion pieces on "Dying with Dignity: A Doctor's and Lawyer's Perspective"; Chochinov & Sneiderman, 2005).[1] In the article, Barney articulated a position he has long held; that is, for those precious few people who would want the option of physician-hastened death, legal means ought to be available. He imagined, however, that this would be a palliative measure of last resort. In the article, he also suggests that no matter how superb the palliative care, there would always be patients who would want to end their lives and his "suspicion" that he would be one of them.

Given this was our final chance to speak, I asked Barney if there was anything he saw or had come to know that he might share with me, from the edge so to speak. He told me that the big surprise of this experience was the fatigue; "like nothing you could ever imagine" were his exact words; "fatigue is the 'f' word in cancer." He told me that he wasn't afraid of death, only the process of getting there, because in the absence of life, there is no experience. He then invoked the words of the Greek philosopher Epicurus: "Where I am, death is not, and where death is, I am not." He went on to say that he was still trying to figure out what death with dignity meant. Without provocation, he suggested that it "may reside with others" (I do not recall ever having given him a copy of my article, "Dignity and the Eye of the Beholder"; Chochinov, 2004).[2] Barney felt his family and friends had showered him with love and attention while he was moving into his final months of life; "the people who come, the food they prepare; they will do anything; and the people in palliative care have been unbelievable; everyone wants to be sure that I don't die alone." Being what he described as an "existentialist," Barney felt that death was an experience he would ultimately face on his own. Although he anticipated his family being by his side, the idea of entering into death alone somehow seemed right and fitting.

He went on to tell me that he still felt there ought to be a legal means by which terminally ill patients could obtain physician-hastened death. He imagined, however, that with good palliative care, this would be exceedingly rare. He described the process being akin to an ancient Hebrew court, where the burden of evidence required was extraordinarily high ("it would practically require a public assassination in front of a dozen witnesses") and the sentence incredibly harsh—death. "And what about you, Barney, is that what you want for yourself?" "No," he replied. "I don't think that would be good for my kids; and so long as I have reassurance that I can be kept comfortable, I'll be OK."

Barney was born on Washington's birthday and had a long-time passion for American and European social, political, and military history. In fact, his final publication will not be the one with our names side by side, but rather, one where his name will stand alone. In his final months of life, he completed a book, *Warriors Seven: Seven American Commanders, Seven Wars and the Irony of Battle*. Like the military leaders he wrote about, in the face of overwhelming odds, he redoubled his efforts to achieve his goal: seeing his book published. Ever the historian, with the official book launch last week, he told me, "June 6th would be a good day to die." June 6th, the most celebrated D-Day of the war, the Allied invasion of Normandy that quickly led to the liberation of northern France. As fate would have it, he died May 28th. He told me he was ready to go, and I know was looking toward death as a liberation from his hard-fought battle with cancer.

As our conversation drew to a close, I think we both sensed it was time to say goodbye, our final goodbye.

"Barney, could I ask you a favor; would you let me write an editorial about you, and share some of our conversations with my palliative care colleagues?"

"I would be honored," he replied. "Harvey, it's been a beautiful thing knowing you."

"It's been a privilege knowing you, Barney."

In his final words to me, Barney said, "This is a strange thing for an atheist to say, but God bless."

At the age of 68, with his wife and three children at his bedside, knowingly embraced in the warmth and affection of multitudes of friends, family, colleagues, and former students, comfortable and at peace, just as he wished, Barney Sneiderman died alone.

References

1. Chochinov HM, Sneiderman B. Dying with dignity: a doctor's and lawyer's perspective. *Canadian Healthcare Manager*. 2005; 12: 23–25. http://www.chmonline.ca/issuearchive/Dec2005/dignity.pdf.
2. Chochinov HM. Dignity and the eye of the beholder. *J Clin Oncol*. 2004;22:1336–1340.

35

Acceptance Speech for Outstanding Achievement in Research Award from the Canadian Cancer Research Alliance

It has been my good fortune to receive various kinds of acknowledgments for my contributions to the field of palliative care. My feelings about these recognitions have evolved over time. When I was starting out, I understood them in terms of affirmation; that is, the universe was telling me what I was doing was good and worthy of praise. With the passage of time, my thinking has changed. While affirmation is nice, it is a bit like popcorn, rapidly consumed and soon forgotten. I now see these professional recognitions in terms of reputational capital—and like most capital, what matters most is how it is spent.

In the early years, reputational capital was spent on personal acquisitions, like a promotion, job security, or a raise. Over time, those things have become less important. This is liberating, allowing reputational capital to be spent more generously. For instance, it can be used to secure resources and opportunities for academics and colleagues wanting to pursue my line of work; it can be used to advocate for and attain services and supports for critically ill patients and their families; and it can be used to elevate the profile and impact of person-centered, dignity-conserving care. This was certainly on my mind during my acceptance speech (delivered from my home on Zoom in the thick of the pandemic) for induction into the Canadian Medical Hall of Fame.

* * * * *

The Canadian Medical Hall of Fame is not something one can ever realistically aspires to. It's a bit like setting one's sites on Pluto; while we know it is somewhere out there in the distant galaxy, it feels impossibly beyond reach. Never in my wildest dreams did I imagine that this achievement was something within my grasp. I am the grandchild of Jewish Russian immigrants who came to this country in and around the time of the Bolshevik Revolution. They arrived in Canada with almost nothing other than the

In Search of Dignity. Harvey Max Chochinov, Oxford University Press. © Oxford University Press 2025.
DOI: 10.1093/9780197805145.003.0035

fervent hope that their children, and their children's children, would find a better life—a life free from persecution, a life where opportunities abound.

Without their vision and sacrifice and my parents' encouragement, I would never have been able to pursue a career in medicine, a career that took me from the University of Manitoba to Memorial Sloan Kettering Cancer Center in New York City, where I gained knowledge and inspiration from the world's leading authorities in neuro-oncology, cancer pain, and psycho-oncology, an area of psychiatry focused on the patient and family experience related to malignant disease. After a few years of working at the Manitoba Cancer Treatment and Research Foundation, I had the good fortune to meet a wonderful psychologist named Keith Wilson, whose guidance and mentorship set me on a course of academic work that, after several decades, has led all the way to Pluto.

My studies in palliative care began by trying to understand what motivates patients to embrace or relinquish their will to live in the face of impending death. This expanded into studies on depression, hopelessness, suicidality, desire for death, and similar topics pertaining to death and dying that my family was never shy to remind me made for horrible dinnertime conversation. Eventually, this led to a program of research on what I coined Dignity Conserving Care, research that has provided insights, set standards of care, and generated outcome measures and therapeutic approaches that have been taken up by palliative care programs worldwide. The essence of dignity is a sense that one continues to have worth regardless of life's circumstances, and hence is deserving of honor, respect, and esteem. The founder of the modern hospice movement, Dame Cicely Saunders, said, "You matter because you are you, and you matter to the end of your life." Supporting or bolstering dignity for those who are dying entails care that acknowledges each patient's continued worth—to never lose sight of the fact that they matter, which means never allowing patienthood to overshadow personhood. In the absence of such care and acknowledgment, patients are bound to suffer as they experience the disintegration of who they are as a person. This can lead to feeling a burden to others, hopelessness, loss of meaning and purpose, and even a desire for early death.

Early into the pandemic I published an article in which I said that "if the first casualty of war is truth, the first casualty of Coronavirus-19 for patients nearing death is human dignity." While the virus has claimed nearly 23,000 lives, in that same time period about 300,000 Canadians have died. Nearly every one of those deaths has been tainted or distorted by this pandemic in some fashion. Patients are required to approach death in isolation, where touch can only be experienced through layers of latex, eye contact through layers of goggles and plastic shields, and human presence through layers of anxiety, caution, and fear. Families are unable to follow a path of least regret, are denied the opportunity to bear witness and advocate for optimal healthcare, and often miss final goodbyes. They are also having to forgo community rituals of mourning. Our healthcare system and those who work in it are also being traumatized, often confronting multiple deaths, moral distress, helplessness, and burnout. Now more than ever, palliative care must help Canadians through this tsunami of suffering, with dignity as a guidepost that will help us find our way.

I am honored to work in a field of medicine that acknowledges our collective humanity and profoundly shapes end-of-life experience. As Victor Frankl said, "Life is never made unbearable by circumstances, but only by lack of meaning and purpose." He went on to say that "those who have a 'why' to live can bear with almost any 'how.'" Professionally, palliative care has given me my "why." Personally, my "why" goes to family: my wife, Michelle; our amazing children, Lauren and Rachel; and my soon-to-be son-in-law Cam. They make the future seem bright and full of wondrous possibilities.

I wish to thank the Canadian Medical Hall of Fame for honoring me beyond anything I ever imagined possible. Pluto is a strange place to arrive. I never expected to be here. I only wish we could have all celebrated my landing, and that of my fellow space traveler inductees, together.

Acceptance Speech for Outstanding Achievement in Research Award from the Canadian Cancer Research Alliance (November 12, 2023, Halifax, Nova Scotia)

Let me clarify what this moment is about.

Today is the culmination of personal events and influences that have made this possible; those who brought me into this world, the family and village of people who raised me; and of course, my wife and children, who stand with me on occasions for celebration, and hold me up in times of sorrow.

The professional pathway leading me here is adorned with mentors, collaborators, and students; I am grateful to them all, and to the granting agencies who, year after year, have supported my work.

But while those influences explain my arrival to this place in time, they are not what this moment is about. Today I share the stage, and this extraordinarily prestigious honour, with one of the world's leading and revered cancer scientists. It would be hubris to suggest my accomplishments are somehow comparable with what my esteemed colleague has contributed to the study of cancer.

However, naming two awardees this year declares to the world, that the areas of study we have devoted ourselves to, are absolutely and undeniably on equal footing. Studying the cellular mysteries of cancer, understanding its biological determinants, and pursuing curative pathways, stand side by side with studying the human experience of cancer; and the ways it affects not only the body, but the mind and the spirit of those afflicted.

Human suffering takes hold in various ways: a cellular aberration, a physical pain, a psychological or spiritual assault, an existential trauma. These are inextricably overlapping and intertwined, with a final common pathway marked by a fractured sense of self; stripping us of our ability to be the person we were, the person we are, or the person we hoped to be. This award, twice given, acknowledges a duality that patients know well; the need to have their malignant ailment addressed, and compassionate caring that safeguards and affirms who they are as people. Today we recognize that complexity, honour that connectivity, and celebrate research that has tried to shed light on the entirety of what it means to have cancer.

36

Address Given to Student Forum, Canadian Medical Hall of Fame

The idea of giving advice to a younger version of myself is intriguing. I was invited to do exactly that with a group of high school students attending a forum organized by the Canadian Medical Hall of Fame. While it was meant to be fun and tongue in cheek, it did get me thinking about words of wisdom and insights accrued over the years.

Love

Love is gentle, love is kind.
Love shows up.
Love doesn't always get its own way.
Love doesn't keep score.
Love experiences giving as restorative.
People who avoid their own feelings will neglect yours.
Love makes you vulnerable, but it's worth it.
Love can hurt, not loving can hurt more.
Walk a path of least regret.

Work

Experience is your greatest teacher.
With time, hard things can get easier and easy things can get harder.
Spend your reputational capital wisely.
Be generous with mentorship; we all start somewhere and need guidance.
Appreciate what work has taught you.
Know there is always more to learn.

In Search of Dignity. Harvey Max Chochinov, Oxford University Press. © Oxford University Press 2025.
DOI: 10.1093/9780197805145.003.0036

Competence and humility can reside on the same page.
Academic success means others will use your achievements to surpass you.
Know your power and use it wisely.
Patients won't care what you know, until they know that you care.
Find joy and meaning in what you do.
Never stop being curious.

Life

Life isn't a dress rehearsal.
Perfectionism is the enemy of the very good.
Much of life is out of our control, so tend to the parts that you can control.
Find a therapist.
Find joy and meaning in the simple things.[a]
Today can't reveal tomorrow's secrets.
Relationships and ideas matter more than things.
With few exceptions, there is always a choice.
Care deeply, intensely, and unashamedly about something.
Power, vitality, and influence are fleeting, so enjoy them while they last.
Vulnerability is woven into the fabric of our existence.
Everyone has their own story; knowing it will open your heart.
While aging diminishes vitality, it does not diminish worth.
The idea of God includes love, connectedness, creativity, and mystery; on that can we agree?

Death

Death is inevitable; suffering ought not to be.
I think it will feel like the time before you were born.
Knowing our days are numbered makes each one more precious.

Address Given to Student Forum, Canadian Medical Hall of Fame. Address given to Student Forum, Canadian Medical Hall of Fame (November 10, 2022, Winnipeg, Manitoba)

---

[a] I recall a woman returning from a day pass in palliative care, telling me about the sheer joy of sitting on her backyard deck, drinking coffee, and feeling the warmth of the sun on her face.

Message to my teenage self...

Harvey, you are going to survive the existential trauma of going bald before the age of 25; it's true, eventually the part in your hair will be as wide as your entire face; and I hate to tell you this, but it will not be the worst thing that ever happens to you, not even by a long shot. Your life will be extraordinary, with highs and lows beyond anything you could ever imagine. The people who love you will be there to celebrate your moments of glory and will also be there to hold you up when you feel unable to do so on your own.

Your time of being a size 28 waist won't last forever. Enjoy eating, sleeping and indulging in various pleasures to your heart's content with equanimity while you can. Life will change and so will you.

A few years from now, you are going to hear about a company called Apple. This has nothing to do with fruit, orchards, or cider. Invest all that you can, as soon as you can, and as much as you can. Trust me, don't ask too many questions, just do it.

You are going to meet some amazing people in the years ahead. Very few, if any of them will try to get in the way of you fulfilling your dreams. You will be your biggest obstacle. Your own self-doubt will cause you to stumble on occasion, more so than anyone else trying to trip you up.

You are going to have the extraordinary privilege of working to make the world a little bit better.

So have faith in the future. Have faith in yourself. Start your hat collection early. And remember, please, please, buy Apple.

37

Address to the Incoming Medical Students, Class of 2028 White Coat Ceremony

Being asked by the Dean of Medicine to deliver the White Coat Ceremony speech for the incoming class of medical students was an honor and a full-circle moment. During the summer of 1977, as I recall, I placed a call to the Faculty of Medicine to make inquiries about entry requirements. The receptionist in the dean's office asked to me identify myself. When I replied "Harvey Chochinov," I was immediately, and to my great surprise, put directly through to the dean!

As it turned out, the dean was expecting a conversation with a different Harvey Chochinov. He assumed the call was from Dr. Harvey Chochinov, a prominent, highly skilled general surgeon practicing at that time. (In response to the question I answered countless times throughout medical school, "Are you two related?", the answer is yes: Dr. Chochinov's father Alex and my great-grandfather Hershel, my namesake, were brothers.) The dean greeted me with a hardy "Hello, Harvey," to which I responded, "I'm looking for information on how to get into medical school." Having realized his error, the conversation ended abruptly.

Surgeon Chochinov had a big personality and a droll sense of humor. He would get annoyed at the occasional mix-ups that were bound to happen. I remember a few years into my practice in outpatient psychiatry being told by my receptionist a patient was in the waiting room "wanting me to perform a cholecystectomy." I gently but firmly impressed on him this wouldn't be a good idea.

Shortly after starting medical school, Harvey Senior, my father Dave, and I found ourselves in conversation at a family gathering.

"We have a real problem," Surgeon Harvey declared.

"What seems to be bothering you, Harvey?" my father asked.

"People keep getting us mixed up."

"Harvey," I said, "I have the perfect and simple solution."

"And what's that?" he said.

In Search of Dignity. Harvey Max Chochinov, Oxford University Press. © Oxford University Press 2025.
DOI: 10.1093/9780197805145.003.0037

"Simple: You need to change your name!"

I did find a wonderful solution. After my paternal grandfather Max Chochinov died, I took on a middle name, thus becoming Harvey Max Chochinov. Max Chochinov was a kind, patient, and wise man. While my feelings about the name Harvey have always been tepid, I associate Max with my Zaida's wonderful characteristics. I've spent much of my professional career studying loss and various dimensions of grief. Part of healing after someone we love dies is finding a way to take them with us. Being Harvey Max Chochinov has allowed me to honor a person who was a role model and inspiration, shaping how I move through life and the values I hold dear.

Address to the Incoming Medical Students, Class of 2028 White Coat Ceremony (August 21, 2024, University of Manitoba, Winnipeg, Manitoba)

Dear Class of 2028:

I am deeply honoured, in the presence of all who have gathered here today, to bear witness as you cross this important threshold into the noble profession of medicine. There are certain inflection points in life; moments that mark a permanent shift; moments that forever alter our course and divide life into before and after. They're sometimes hard to spot when they are actually happening. But trust me, this is one such moment. Years from now, or even decades from now, you'll look back and see that today marked the beginning of what I hope will be a long, productive and meaningful career in the field of medicine.

For some of you—considering the time, the work, and the longing that preceded your arrival here today—this moment may seem surreal. But remember, you've earned your place in the class of 2028. No one handed it to you. Study, dedication and ability got you here; and study, dedication and ability will propel you along the most life changing, pedagogical adventure you could ever imagine.

But before I describe that journey, let me say that the quality of education you will receive at the University of Manitoba is second to none (the dean did not ask me to say this). It has been my good fortune to lecture and teach in places whose names are steeped in history, tradition, and drip with status; places like Harvard, Yale, Cornell, Stanford, The University of Oxford, King's

College, Cambridge, and the list covers hundreds of others across the entire globe. I can tell you, having seen it firsthand, the quality of students and the quality of instructors here at home take a back seat to none of them. Which means receiving your MD at the Max Rady College of Medicine will set you up for whatever you want to do in any capacity, here at home or anywhere on earth.

As for the journey itself, because of its sheer complexity, you will be guided along what at times will feel like multiple parallel pathways. Cardiology, neurology, nephrology, rheumatology, respirology, endocrinology, immunology, hepatology, gastroenterology, ophthalmology, otolaryngology and various other 'ology's' that are sure to keep you busy and fully engaged over the next four years. While this *siloing* of the human body is necessary to help you wrap your mind around its various complexities, there is a danger, and that is losing sight of the whole person. In my own writings, I describe this as the problem of patienthood eclipsing personhood.

I recall a mid-career dialysis nurse telling me she felt burnt out. "After so many years," she said, "patients have begun to feel like kidneys on legs." She knew this wasn't good for her, nor her patients or their families, because it meant she no longer saw them as whole persons. Our research shows when this happens, it can diminish trust, empathy, compassion and respect. Patients who don't feel seen are less likely to trust us, or to tell us what they really need, increasing the chances of discordance in goals of care. Our studies also show when healthcare providers experience patients based solely on their illness, without consideration for who these patients are as persons, they become less satisfied with their jobs, more robotic in their work, and more vulnerable to burnout.

Another interesting thing we found was that "how patients perceive themselves to be seen" is the strongest predictor of sense of dignity. In other words, patients are looking for a reflection in the eye of the healthcare provider that will affirm their sense of themselves. If all they see in this metaphorical reflection is a problem check list or a differential diagnosis, they end up feeling that the essence of who they are as a person has fallen off our clinical radar. This idea of personhood being under assault, or threatened, or starting to disintegrate, has long been considered central to the experience of human suffering.

So, we must ask patients what they would want known about them as persons to provide them the best care possible. Take it from me, the responses you will get to that question will permanently change the way you see your patients. A former head of a department of medicine told me, while being treated for cancer, that he felt like a pip—PIP—previously important person. When I asked an Aboriginal woman with advanced cancer on our ward what I should know about her as a person, she told me she was a residential school survivor, that her family had moved 82 times so no one would know them, and that she didn't trust healthcare professionals who wore white coats. Without knowing something so central about who people are and the nature of their suffering, a commitment to person-centered care is little more than lip service.

What all of this means is the way we are with patients and our attitude towards them, will profoundly shape every single clinical encounter and their illness experience. This means you need to be mindful of your outlook, and more specifically, what shapes it. We all intuitively tend to use ourselves as a gauge for what patients want or need; the so-called Golden Rule; doing unto others as we'd want done unto ourselves. This is an important moral adage, appearing in various religious traditions across millennia. But we need to be aware that the lens through which we see our patients has been shaped in ways we may not be entirely aware of.

About five years before she died, my sister Ellen was back in hospital, this time in intensive care. Ellen was born with cerebral palsy and had many of the physical challenges that go along with that condition, including poor respiratory capacity because of various complex anatomical distortions. She couldn't blow out her birthday candles, which by the end of her life numbered 55, if her life depended on it. But this admission to ICU was unlike any other, because she was now on the brink of respiratory collapse, and the question of intubation was on the table. I remember her intensivist pacing the unit, as he contemplated whether she would need a breathing tube inserted. At one point, he came over to ask me the only question he'd asked about personhood: "Does she read magazines"? It struck me as an odd question, and it took a minute or so to sink in. His unspoken question was "is this the kind of person we should be intubating?" He could see her bent spine; he could see her spastic limbs; he could see her dropping blood gases. What he couldn't see was Ellen, and the rich, full, complex life she lived. Realizing her life hung in the balance, I took a deep breath and said, "Yes, she can read magazines. But only when she's in between novels."

Amongst Ellen's problems that day, besides her difficulties breathing, was the lens of the healthcare provider, through which he could only see her suffering. I can assure you, when she was on the dance floor, the only people who suffered were those whose toes she crushed, unapologetically, under the massive weight of her electric wheelchair.

The take home lesson is, the Golden Rule must accommodate what I have coined the Platinum Rule, which would have us *doing unto others as they would want done unto themselves.* This is a reminder that we must face our own biases and have the humility to know we can't presume to understand how someone sees and experiences their life and their priorities.

I mentioned earlier you might be finding this ceremony rather surreal; I forgot to say those feelings apply to me as well. My medical education began 46 years ago, in 1978 (yes, Trudeau was still Prime Minister, and yes, my daughter warned me the younger members in the audience might not get that particular humour). While I hear myself saying these words aloud, it seems inconceivable that nearly half a century has slipped by. Trust me, while the days may seem to move slowly—and you find yourself thinking that some clinical rotations will never end—the years go by in a flash.

After my first 10 years in practice, I felt I could claim professional credibility. Twenty years in, I had become what you might describe as a seasoned clinician. Three decades later, people started to use words like *senior* scientist, *distinguished* professor, and *pioneer*. While I know those were always spoken in kindness, they did imply I was moving—ever so gently but steadily—towards my "best before" date. And now, closing in on five decades has me thinking that destiny may see me become a "fading faculty fossil." But so far, those who sign my contract have seen fit to keep me around.

So let me close with some advice, flavoured with a fossil-like perspective.

1. The past is irretrievable, and tomorrow is uncertain and unknowable. The only thing you can absolutely know is the here and now. So be present in your life. Take in today, and each subsequent today you are fortunate enough to be given. Take in the privilege of learning and evolving; of love and relationships and experiences; and take time to express gratitude to those who make you covet more tomorrows.

2. Resist comparing yourself with others. Self-doubt may find you thinking others are more capable than you; are smarter than you, are more deserving than you. But consider this; since the beginning of time, 117 billion people have been born on Earth, and never has there been (nor will there ever again be) one entirely like you. Each of you belong here, and each of you bring talent, experiences, perspectives, creative and intellectual energies that are entirely unique. That is

something you should honour and nurture. Allow yourself to dream and pursue whatever goals you are striving to attain. Make peace with the person who looks back at you in the mirror each day. If you can do that, you'll be able to work out your connections with everyone else.

3. Strive to be more than human-body mechanics. Aspire to be healers. Years ago, I wrote an article called, "The Secret's Out: Patients are People with Feelings that Matter." You are about to spend years looking at your books; and will soon be spending years, looking at clinical charts. But I implore you to look up from those books and charts, and to see your patients. Patients will not care what you know, until they know that you care.

4. Making connections with patients based on caring—what I call the human side of medicine—will infuse your work with meaning and purpose and richness, which will nurture and sustain you over the course of your entire career.

5. Resist scepticism and despair. There is no shortage of pain and conflict in the world. Life can be hard. Working in medicine will expose you to situations that will sometimes make you feel there is no justice, nor rhyme or reason for the suffering people must endure. As healers, you aren't expected to cure what can't be cured, or fix what can't be fixed. But you are expected to show up for your patients; to accompany them. Please know that in exercising kindness and compassion in every clinical encounter, with every person whose path you cross, you are playing your small part in bending the arc of the universe towards hope, healing and peace.

Class of 2028. Welcome to the profession of medicine; a profession William Osler, one of the great pioneers in our field, described as "the science of uncertainty and the art of probabilities." While no one can say with certainty where medicine will take you, the possibilities are limitless. Enjoy this magnificent, transformative journey; and use all you learn along the way to make the world a better place.

Index

For the benefit of digital users, indexed terms that span two pages (e.g., 52–53) may, on occasion, appear on only one of those pages.

Page numbers followed by *f* and *t* indicate figures and tables, respectively.